THE BEACH CURE

WEYERHAEUSER ENVIRONMENTAL BOOKS

Paul S. Sutter, Editor

Weyerhaeuser Environmental Books explore human relationships with natural environments in all their variety and complexity. They seek to cast new light on the ways that natural systems affect human communities, the ways that people affect the environments of which they are a part, and the ways that different cultural conceptions of nature profoundly shape our sense of the world around us. A complete list of the books in the series appears at the end of this book.

MEGHAN CRNIC

the BEACH CURE

A History of Healing on Northeastern Shores

University of Washington Press *Seattle*

The Beach Cure is published with the assistance of a grant from the Weyerhaeuser Environmental Books Endowment, established by the Weyerhaeuser Company Foundation, members of the Weyerhaeuser family, and Janet and Jack Creighton.

Design by Mindy Basinger Hill

Composed in Adobe Jenson Pro

UNIVERSITY OF WASHINGTON PRESS *uwapress.uw.edu*

Cataloging information is available from the Library of Congress

LIBRARY OF CONGRESS CONTROL NUMBER 2024053086
ISBN 9780295753942 (hardcover)
ISBN 9780295753959 (paperback)
ISBN 9780295753966 (ebook)

∞ This paper meets the requirements of ANSI/NISO Z39.48-1992 (Permanence of Paper).

TO TIM, JACK, AND JOHN

Whose health and love I am grateful for every day

CONTENTS

ix Foreword: The Salubrious Seashore, by Paul S. Sutter

xv Acknowledgments

1 Introduction

9 Chapter 1. Cities and the Pathology of Place

35 Chapter 2. Finding Cures at the Shore

58 Chapter 3. The Shifting Sands of Health Tourism

79 Chapter 4. How Working-Class Mothers Shaped the Shore

97 Chapter 5. Pediatric Patients at the Beach

123 Chapter 6. Doctor Sun and Technologies of Nature

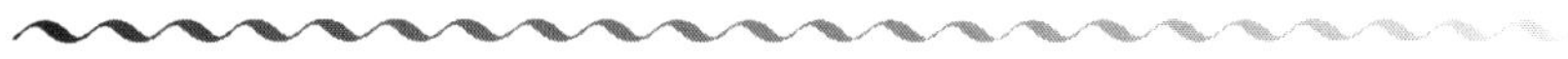

143 Conclusion

153 Notes

177 Bibliography

195 Index

FOREWORD The Salubrious Seashore *Paul S. Sutter*

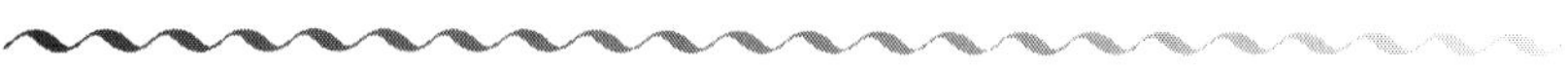

LET'S ADMIT IT: the beach is a weird place. Americans are eager beachgoers, and beaches are often our preferred vacation destinations. Indeed, the authors of a recent article in *Shore & Beach*, the peer-reviewed journal of the American Shore and Beach Preservation Association, estimate that roughly half of the US population visits a beach at least once per year and that US beaches collectively experience 3.4 *billion* annual visits. That is a staggering number, more than ten times the 325.5 million visits to the four hundred National Park Service units that reported annual visitation numbers in 2023. And that's not counting those Americans with means who travel the globe searching out pristine beaches with posh amenities or the beach-going public in the rest of the world. Once we get to these beaches, we swim, yes, but we also loll on towels and blankets in the sand (abiding its annoyances), recline in beach chairs while soaking up the sun and salty sea air, and happily watch children frolic in the surf. We do all these things on the verge of nudity, as few other spaces allow for such a relaxation of the rules around what it means to be properly clothed in public. Beaches are also magnets for other sorts of entertainment, from amusement parks and resorts to nightclubs and casinos. And despite abundant evidence of the dangers of doing so in a warming world, we continue to build along beaches, the proximity of surf and sand numbing us to the risks of doing so. What is the allure of the beach as an environment of recreation and relaxation? And why have environmental historians paid so little attention to this important natural and cultural space?

The human love affair with the beach has not been a timeless one. In the Western world prior to the eighteenth century, most people saw beaches as hostile and desolate, as all-but-empty spaces save for the scattered communities of fisher folk hauling in a living from an unforgiving sea. But as scholars such as Alain Corbin and Robert C. Ritchie have shown, something changed in the eighteenth and nineteenth centuries. Artists and writers began to see the seashore as a romantic and sublime space, as they had done with other environments, such as mountains. And as scientists took to the shore to collect natural history specimens and contemplate the oceans' mysteries, they too gave new value to beaches. These developments were shaped in turn by other historical trends that fed the growth of nature appreciation: urbanization, industrialization, the rise of a leisure class, and the proliferation of railroads and other modes of transportation that provided easy access to distant environments. The beach as we know it was thus a modern invention, our strange beach-going habits the product of a specific set of historical circumstances. To understand the allure of the beach, we need to know that history.

But there was another reason why we began to flock to the beach. As Meghan Crnic demonstrates in *The Beach Cure*, her elegant history of beach-going along the northeastern US coast, the allure of the beach was also therapeutic, rooted in the claims of medical professionals and entrepreneurs who made the "beach cure" a common prescription for those suffering from a panoply of diseases and debilities in the nineteenth and early twentieth centuries. Such therapeutic claims originated in Europe, leading to the early development of beach resorts there, but they soon spread across the Atlantic to the United States. Not surprisingly, these claims built on more venerable ones made for the healing powers of mineral springs, but the beach cure developed its own environmental therapeutics across the nineteenth century. Indeed, it was part of a larger movement in which Americans traveled to supposedly salubrious environments—the piney woods of the South, the forests of New England and the upper Midwest, the Colorado Front Range, the deserts of the Southwest, and "semitropical" Southern California—to seek health. Environment and health were inextricably linked in nineteenth-century America.

The rise of the beach cure was also part and parcel of the massive transformations remaking the nation's urban environments. During the nineteenth century, as populations grew in places like Philadelphia, New York, and Boston, and as those cities became increasingly polluted, residents experienced growing problems with disease. For many doctors and reformers, industrial cities were unnatural places, and they focused particularly on the well-being of children, who seemed to be acutely susceptible to urban diseases. Crnic reveals for us how deadly the nation's cities had become for children across the nineteenth century, with infant mortality rates as high as 25 to 30 percent and widespread respiratory, intestinal, and nutritional diseases debilitating children. Physicians worried that cramped living conditions, the lack of fresh air and clean water, and the paucity of safe places for children to play amounted to an urban public health crisis. One response was to reform the urban environment and particularly to provide more parks and playgrounds scattered throughout these cities. Tellingly, one early form of urban recreation was the sand garden, which provided sandboxes or sandpiles for children to play in, bringing a little bit of the beach into the city. But another response was to move sick and debilitated children out of polluted cities, particularly during the hot summer months. It was in this context that the beaches of the northeastern seaboard took on new therapeutic importance.

While the well-to-do pioneered the therapeutic beach retreat, the practice soon spread to those of lower status, thanks to a series of charities and seaside institutions that catered to the poor and working classes. *The Beach Cure* is particularly innovative in its focus on the histories of these institutions and the experiences of the working-class women and children to whom they catered. Such children and their mothers initially went to the shore under the wings of physicians and reformers, but they soon made claims of their own on the beach cure. Crnic provides a fascinating history of the seaside houses, floating hospitals, and mothers' cottages that dotted the coast and of the women and children who were their clients. Children frequented these institutions to receive treatment for a wide variety of ailments, while mothers often claimed these retreats as well-earned vacations from grinding domestic routines. "Pediatric seashore hospitals and health homes gave urban mothers a place to breathe, literally and figuratively," Crnic notes, and in so doing they empowered these women to define the experience as one of both health and leisure.

One thing that doctors and patients agreed upon was the efficacy of the beach cure. Children who went to the beach sickly and pallid usually returned home with rosy cheeks and meat on their bones, and the beach seemed to work wonders for those suffering from more serious conditions such as rickets, tuberculosis, or persistent diarrhea. For young patients and their families, the seashore was a self-evidently salubrious environment, and their experiences of healing contributed in important ways to scientific knowledge production about the beach. But as physicians tried to make sense of the curative powers of the beach, Crnic argues, they were so eager to pinpoint the sources of nature's therapeutic efficacy that they eroded our ability to see and know the environment's ability to heal.

Physicians focused on three aspects of the beach environment that seemed particularly healing: fresh sea breezes, salt water, and sunshine. Soon they isolated these elements from the environment as a whole and rendered them in the argot of medical expertise, as balneotherapy (swimming) and heliotherapy (sunbathing), for instance, carefully dosing each of these distinctive elements. In terms of our contemporary medical understandings of the causes of these diseases, these specific elements of the beach likely were curative. In the case of rickets, for instance, medical researchers in the years after World War I came to recognize vitamin D deficiency as its cause, and one source of vitamin D is sunlight. Children growing up in crowded, windowless tenements in cities where air pollution often blotted out the sun were thus particularly susceptible to rickets, and the sunshine (and improved diet) that came with a stay at a seaside hospital surely had a salutary effect. But Crnic is careful not to impose our contemporary understandings of these diseases on the past, instead asking us to see the continuing value in the more holistic environmental therapeutics of the era.

The beach cure was at the leading edge of Americans' growing recreational enthusiasm for the beach vacation, but as the twentieth century progressed, the therapeutic origins of the beach retreat dropped from public discourse. Part of the problem was the reductiveness of modern medicine, as practitioners distilled the curative properties of the beach and then imported them into urban clinical settings. UV lamps replaced sunbathing, saline solutions mimicked the effects of sea bathing, and scientists isolated ozone as the curative feature of sea air. This is a familiar story in the literature on health and the environment, a story in which modern medicine abandoned environmental approaches and medical therapies became placeless. As Crnic aptly puts it,

"The more physicians sought to rationalize the marine environment, the harder it became to conceptualize the seashore as holistically salubrious." In the process, the beach became less a place of healing and more a place of recreation. In one of the most vivid symbols of this transition, Crnic suggests, the wheelchairs that had been a prominent part of Atlantic City's therapeutic landscape were repurposed into rolling chairs—instruments of tourist entertainment. But Crnic is not quite ready to see an irrevocable turn from health to leisure, or from nature to technology. Rather, hers is a story in which health and leisure claims became melded into a potent new amalgam and the beach's therapeutic environmental qualities remained, though increasingly invisible and unrecognized.

It would be all too easy to dismiss the health claims of those who boosted beaches and "marine medication" at the turn of the last century as vague, exaggerated, or unscientific, and, indeed, historians have tended to neglect this medical history of the beach for precisely these reasons. But Crnic insists that it would be a mistake to do so. *The Beach Cure* joins a growing list of important books on how people historically understood and experienced the natural world through their bodily well-being and how they produced meaningful scientific knowledge in the process. These historians have insisted, as Crnic does, that the lens of health was crucial to American environmental thinking before the advent of germ theory, and they lament the twentieth-century retreat from such environmental understandings of disease and health as limiting the efficacy of modern medicine. *The Beach Cure*, then, is not only a history of how we once valued the beach as a restorative environment but also a prescription for rethinking how we currently understand its value, as well as the value of other place-based therapeutic approaches.

We are now living in a new era of purported environmental therapies, though proponents of these contemporary "nature fixes" often seem more interested in the effects of the natural world on our mental rather than our physical well-being. Unlike a century or more ago, they focus more on sanity than sanitation. Yet we still speak of seashore vacations as recuperative and restorative; physicians increasingly turn to "nature prescriptions" to help their patients reduce rising levels of stress, anxiety, and depression; and "nature deficit disorder" has become a particular concern when it comes to the health of America's children, who, like their peers in the late nineteenth and early twentieth centuries, seem dangerously cut off from the sunshine and fresh air of the outdoors. Modern medicine has even come around to recognizing that a trip to the beach might have curative properties, as Crnic reveals in her surprising conclusion. These contemporary diagnoses of environmental disconnection might seem new, but they have strong resonances with the environmental therapies of the late nineteenth and early twentieth centuries. By illuminating the hidden origins of our weird affection for sun, surf, and salty air, *The Beach Cure* is a wonderful historical guide to this new moment, a book that insists that the boundaries between health and recreation, bodies and environments, have never been as clear as we have thought them to be.

ACKNOWLEDGMENTS

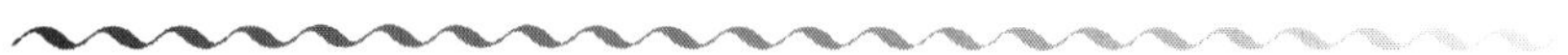

ACKNOWLEDGMENTS ARE OFTEN my favorite part of academic books. They are a rare moment when we are gifted a glimpse into the lives of authors. I am awed by the task of finally writing my own. I cannot adequately acknowledge everyone who touched these pages. If you can count yourself among this group, please know that my appreciation for you is vast.

I want to begin with the people closest to the project, because they are closest to me: my family. My sons, Tim and Jack, have always known their mom was working on a research project about the beach and have been incredible company as we traveled to the Jersey shore, Cape Cod, and beyond. They are a source of constant joy, perspective, grounding, and growth. My husband, John, has read every chapter (too) many times. His unwavering presence and support have inspired me to persist. John, thank you for copiloting and for taking on more than your fair share of the domestic duties of late.

A corps of caregivers made raising two humans possible while writing this book. I am grateful to the many women who loved, nurtured, and taught my kids. In particular, Ashley and Narci, I hold you both in my heart. I am also blessed with an amazing group of friends who still ask with genuine interest how my book is going. Thank you for loving food, travel, and exploring Philadelphia as much as I do. You keep me balanced and well fed.

To my parents, who often made us visit historic sites: I know we complained, but those experiences are clearly woven into the fabric of our being. Mom, thanks for exposing us to American history; Dad, thanks for making sure our road trips included amusement parks; and Allison, thanks for sharing activities like lawn bowling in Williamsburg, chasing wooden hoops with sticks in Sturbridge, and dressing up in period garb with me. I am also fortunate to have amazing in-laws who once, after hearing me talk about my research, interrupted a neighboring diner to tell them that they should forgo a swimming pool and visit the beach instead. Eileen and Joe, thank you for your support and spreading the word.

To my students: you are inspiring. What a gift and privilege to be in the classroom with you! I was fortunate to work with two of the most exceptional, intelligent, and generous women as research assistants. Natalie Doppelt and Camryn Harvie, your depth of knowledge, keen minds, and bright spirits infused the writing process with joy when I needed it most.

Innumerable colleagues, friends, and advisers have been by my side as I wrote. You come from all points of my professional development: graduate school, my work at Penn, Drexel, Columbia, and Cooper Medical School at Rowan University. If you ever took the time to talk, listen, or read some version of this along the way, thank you. I have also been fortunate to have many mentors who have shaped me as a scholar. Karen-Sue Taussig, you inspired me to pursue a career in academics and have continued to guide me. For this book in particular, Conevery Bolton Valenčius, Cindy Connolly, and Beth Linker: I appreciate the time and your generative and productive feedback over the years. Michael Yudell, your encouragement inspired me to see this project through.

Melanie Kiechle and Elaine LaFay, my friends, writing partners, and support system: thank you for your unwavering friendship and belief in this book. You are shining examples of how generous environmental historians are to one another. I want to give special praise to Paul Sutter and everyone at the University of Washington Press for their steadfast commitment to this project. This book is much richer given the honest and constructive perspectives from you and my anonymous reviewers, and I appreciate all the time you donated to this project. And a special thanks to Katherine Carroll and Maureen Bemko, exceptional editors whose gifts with the English language are awesome.

As most historians will attest, archivists and librarians are too often unsung heroes, so here is a special shout out to the folks at the College of Physicians, Historical Society of Pennsylvania, the Boston Floating Hospital, St. Christopher's Hospital, Countway Library at Harvard Medical School, and the

Philadelphia and Atlantic City public libraries for their assistance over the years. And thank you to the Consortium for History of Science, Technology, and Medicine; the Barbara Bates Center for the Study of the History of Nursing, University of Pennsylvania; and the M. Louise Carpenter Gloeckner, M.D., Summer Research Fellowship from the Drexel University College of Medicine Archives and Special Collections on Women in Medicine for financially supporting my research.

To Howard Gershenfeld's family, thank you for trusting me with your father's story. I hope I have done him justice.

Dr. Ed Viner: you are not here to read these words, but every day I am grateful you took my call and took a chance by hiring me, a historian. To my colleagues at the Center for Humanism: thank you for welcoming me into your fold. What an honor to work with whip-smart and compassionate physicians.

Finally, thank you to my readers. Thank you for picking up this book and for supporting scholarship. Thank you for being curious enough to peruse the pages that follow. I hope you find that *The Beach Cure* inspires you to think about the spaces and places we travel and that it gives you hope that there are other ways of knowing and experiencing our surroundings. Maybe this book helps you think differently about your time at the beach with family and friends and explains why you always want that extra ice cream. Time at the beach awakens the appetite; I hope this book leaves you satisfied.

THE BEACH CURE

INTRODUCTION

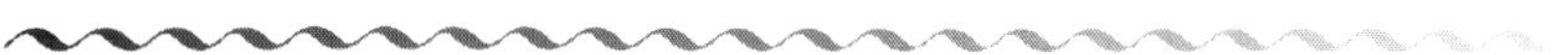

BEACH VACATIONS should be counterintuitive. We bring babies and young children who cannot swim to a place where seas swell, waves crash, and undertows can whisk even the strongest swimmers out to open water. We hop over scalding sand to stake a small space among scores of strangers, a group we otherwise condition children to think of as potentially dangerous. We bathe bodies beneath the bright sun that toasts us in the short term and possibly causes cancer in the future. Children play in sand that can swallow and even bury them alive.[1]

Few people question the wisdom of this annual migration, but beach excursions are a recent phenomenon. For centuries the Western world looked at the ocean with suspicion, associating it with work, exploration, exploitation, and danger.[2] It was only in the early nineteenth century that a few wealthy Americans ventured to seaside perches, seeking an escape from the summertime heat and its incumbent diseases.[3] What started as a trickle of tourists turned into a torrent over the next one hundred years. By 1900, millions of tourists flocked to the northeastern shores of the United States every summer, making the beach one of the most popular vacation destinations.[4]

Today we think of the beach as a place of rest, leisure, and pleasure, but Americans also used to view the seashore as a therapeutic landscape.[5] In the nineteenth century, and continuing into the twentieth, doctors prescribed trips to the beach, and patients eagerly took what one French physician termed "marine medication."[6] In the United States, people across social and professional spectrums embraced the beach as a site of health and healing. Trains shuttled patients and tourists between American cities and their nearby shorelines, while physicians and nurses at seaside hospitals cared for urban children.[7]

Working-class families took advantage of the health care institutions, applying for admission at rates that outstripped hospitals' capacity. Sick children might stay in a hospital, while those who were merely run-down visited health homes that philanthropic groups built to serve the urban masses.[8] Wealthier families could rent rooms at newly built hotels, while the most fortunate owned private cottages or houses. Regardless of financial or health status, most Americans agreed that they benefited from time at the beach.

This book uncovers the therapeutic origins of US seashores and traces how physicians, tourists, and urban families changed this environment and its meanings over time. It shows how and why in the mid- to late nineteenth century Americans imagined that vast expanses of open shoreline could cure and physically reform droves of weary, sick, and dying urban children and their caregivers. Readers will discover that health professionals shared ideologies with working-class urban mothers, children, and wealthier tourists about the interconnections between bodies, well-being, and place.

We will see that Americans who sought health also found leisure at the beach.[9] This new paradigm shifted cultural associations about the seashore and resulted in significant alterations to the built environment. This is not, however, a history of straightforward environmental degradation. It is, at its heart, an exploration of how Americans viewed their health as enmeshed with their environments and understood that places shaped their bodies. The chapters that follow uncover how these ideas persisted across incredible social and cultural divides and medical changes.

Critically, *The Beach Cure* argues that neither physicians nor tourists ever rejected the belief that the seashore was therapeutic. Rather, Americans' changing ideas reflected and reinforced a growing transformation in how people understood that specific places, climates, and landscapes could reform bodies and restore health. These shifts left voids that Americans filled with leisure and pleasure pursuits. It is a legacy that remains today.

The Beach Cure is situated along the northeastern seaboard of the United States in the decades around the turn of the twentieth century because this was a time and place of seismic environmental, medical, social, and cultural change. At this time, the US population was concentrating in the region that stretched from Baltimore, Maryland, to Boston, Massachusetts. The intertwined processes of industrialization and immigration had resulted in rapid urban growth. As people poured into the cities from the countryside and from overseas to work in factories that darkened the skies, they witnessed the environmental deterioration of the urban landscape.[10]

Filthy conditions led public health commissioners to sniff out the sources of various diseases, especially as epidemics ravaged urban populations. Plagues of yellow fever, cholera, diphtheria, and infantile paralysis (polio) swept through cities and claimed scores of lives.[11] Children were particularly susceptible. Parents learned that nearly one in four children born in cities would die before celebrating their first birthday. While some babies perished during epidemics, many more succumbed to diarrheal diseases that were particularly deadly during the summer. Statistics quantified what people had long known—that cities stole health.

Yet nineteenth-century urban residents and health professionals did not need statistics to prove that cities were pathological places. Their noses warned them of these dangers every day. Before the 1880s, ideas about miasmas dominated notions about health and disease. Medical and popular belief held that bodies absorbed the noxious fumes emanating from rotting material, resulting in illness and death. Although city governments began public health efforts to improve sanitation, privies abounded and residents tossed kitchen scraps into alleys.[12] Livestock roamed about, eating debris and contributing their own, while horses clip-clopped down the streets, leaving trails of excrement.[13] The resulting stench assaulted not only noses but also residents' bodies, health, and well-being.[14] Smells equaled disease, and cities stank.[15]

While nineteenth-century medical conceptualizations differed from those of today, they were not unsophisticated or misguided. Instead, people maintain different ways of knowing that conform to prevailing medical wisdom and scientific evidence.[16] If we inquire and accept that the ideas made sense within their time and place, it opens new ways of understanding historical actors' logic and decision-making. It can even allow us to question how similar forces shape our contemporary ideas and practices.

Just as urban environments experienced massive upheaval around the turn of the twentieth century, so too did American medicine. By the 1880s, physicians had begun to embrace germ theory, which shifted notions of disease etiology from the environment to microscopic germs, including bacteria. Germ theory gave birth to a legion of microbe hunters, sending researchers, scientists, and physicians scurrying between the laboratory and the field in a search for bacteriologic causes and vectors. A few new and exciting discoveries followed, among them vaccines for anthrax and rabies, an antitoxin for diphtheria, and the discovery that mosquitoes were vectors for diseases, including yellow fever.[17]

Despite these changes, neither the American public nor the country's medical practitioners lost faith in nature's ability to cure. Historians have examined how older environmental ideologies intermingled with new notions of microscopic agents, even as physicians ceased to identify environmental culprits as the agents of disease.[18] Moreover, while germ theory pinpointed the cause of illness, most so-called magic-bullet treatments—a single pill that could cure a specific disease—remained decades in the future.

More importantly, germ theory said almost nothing about how to promote health, restore well-being, or rebuild bodies broken down by disease and urban life.[19] This void allowed people to continue to believe that landscapes, like the seashore, could provide patients with efficacious health care and cures. Understanding the environmental, medical, and social changes also helps us analyze how Americans came to idealize their shores in direct response to concerns about city life.

Americans had long used their bodies as barometers for the health of a place.[20] If you were sick in one location, traveling to another could result in better health. Doctors sent patients suffering from hay fever, asthma, and tuberculosis to the mountains for a dose of fresh air.[21] Although the rise of laboratory-based medical science in the late nineteenth century gradually dislodged older environmental notions of the causes of disease, it did not dissuade Americans from a persistent belief that natural environments were superior to the city. Indeed, patients suffering from tuberculosis continued to travel to sanatoriums in the mountains into the mid-twentieth century, when antibiotics provided a targeted cure.

The idea that nature could be healthy has deep roots. As historians have argued, nature is a messy category, with definitions that shift over time.[22] In the nineteenth and early twentieth centuries, Americans often defined nature as environments untouched by humans, or as green spaces, fresh air, and sunshine. If nature was healthy and cities lacked open spaces, it made sense that one should head for the less developed and less congested country, mountains, or seashore.[23]

Physicians who recommended travel for health rhapsodized about the curative powers of nature. However, their conceptualizations differed from those of boosters who crowed about the vast, untamed landscapes that instilled travelers with moral, religious, and physical well-being.[24] The expansiveness of the ocean must have inspired awe among some tourists, but practitioners and patients alike focused on how environments, especially one's immediate surroundings, impacted large groups of travelers' health and well-being.[25] Moreover, the spaces along the United States' northeastern shores quickly developed into popular tourist attractions, replete with carnivalesque rides that competed with the natural environment for travelers' time. Going to those popular health resorts in the summer months could require standing elbow to elbow with fellow tourists along the boardwalk or shimmying into a narrow space on a busy beach.[26] It was a far cry from the romantic imaginations of the lone figure standing atop a mountain.

While different from the breathtaking vistas of the American West, large bodies of water beckoned weary urban residents. Those dwelling in landlocked cities such as Chicago and Toronto used the Great Lakes, while residents who lived along the northeastern corridor looked to the ocean.[27] The open expanses of shoreline provided fresh air and a fresh start. With fewer buildings or people, cool breezes swirled, the sun shone, and waves lapped the sands. They were the smells, sights, and sounds of salubrity. By the early 1900s, millions of Americans were taking advantage of the beach as a landscape of health and leisure.

In the chapters that follow we will travel with different patrons as they move between the city and the shore. This approach will allow us to explore the ways in which various parties, from visitors to developers, effectively built a new physical landscape, as well as to discern the broader cultural conceptions of the seashore and its meanings. The chapters are thematic, a structure that enables deeper interrogation of how specific groups' actions and beliefs converged. Disentangling these narratives, and then tracing historical threads within chapters, provides a comprehensive view of changes that occurred over time.

We begin in urban centers, including Philadelphia, New York, and Boston. We examine what life was like there, how residents constructed ideas regarding the pathologic effects of cities, and why Americans understood that children were particularly vulnerable to cities' insalubrious forces. Understanding the urban condition that working-class families endured makes it easy to see why people would want to escape to the seashore.

It is more confounding that physicians prescribed so-called marine medication even into the twentieth century, given the paradigmatic shifts in medical ideologies. We will learn that physicians documented the seashore's salubrious effects on a vast range of medical conditions. Although germ theory did little to diminish doctors' conviction that environments could be curative, it did inspire them to use laboratory-based methods to establish quantifiable and measurable evidence of impact. This shift gradually inhibited medical professionals' ability to see the holistic effects of the seashore on patients' bodies. Physicians' vision became increasingly myopic, but tourists and patients continued to fill their seashore prescriptions.

We will then turn to middle- and upper-class tourists, who consumed and quickly transformed health care practices and technologies, including bathhouses and wheelchairs, into vehicles of leisure. Their activities may have been rooted in health, but their behaviors transformed medical interventions into pleasurable pursuits. Next, we turn our attention to working-class mothers, a group that has received far less attention in the history of tourism.[28] Not only were these women savvy consumers of seaside health practices, but they also established the shoreline as a space of pleasure that was appropriate for all social classes.[29] Children occupy the final group under study. While they leave few written records, they were consequential actors who altered and were shaped by the places they lived, worked, played, and healed.[30] When children traveled to the beach, they reinforced notions that the seashore was a space of play and pleasure, as well as health and healing.

Studying these actors allows us to trace how their experiences and per-

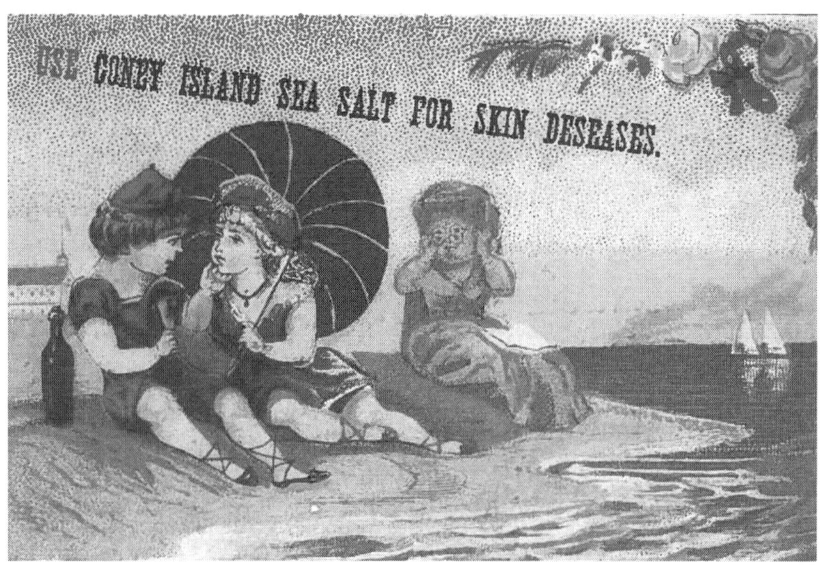

FIGURE 1. Advertisement for Coney Island Sea Salt, probably late nineteenth century. Image of two young children sitting on beach. The reverse side highlights the salt's medical properties and its strengthening effects on children. Author's collection.

ceptions changed over time and transformed the northeastern seaboard of the United States from a place of health to one primarily associated with leisure and entertainment. The final chapter turns our gaze to technologies that seemingly supplanted marine medication. Using the UV lamp as a case study helps us understand one reason why Americans are no longer able to medically explain the therapeutic influence of the seashore. We will learn that physicians constructed technologies to support their belief that sunlight could cure. Ironically, if unsurprisingly, the embrace of devices like UV lamps, or of products like saline solution and Coney Island Sea Salt, made it easier for patients to stay in cities for treatment. Technologies mediated bodies and natural environments and rendered places like the seashore medically unnecessary.

Over the twentieth century, Americans may have lost sight of the beach as a therapeutic landscape, but practices that began as health prescriptions in the nineteenth century continue today. This book offers a way to understand why we jam our families into cars, which we pack full of towels, trowels, buckets, and bathing suits, and head to the seashore. It provides new perspectives of why we bring babies to the beach, bob in the waves, and bask under the sun. When we do, we are connecting with a set of practices rooted in historical understanding that the seashore is healing.

My hope is that *The Beach Cure* provides us with new ways of thinking about our bodies and place, that it will give us insight into why some people report they feel better at the seashore but lack a medical lexicon to describe their embodied experiences. We might express our feelings in terms of relaxation, rest, or wellness but not as curative, therapeutic, and preventive health care. Uncovering the origins of seaside vacations as a search for health, and tracing how Americans transformed their shorelines, enables us to see how the choices we make have profound consequences for human and environmental health. *The Beach Cure* offers a reminder that it is possible to have profound and rapid impact on the environment, to knit together human and environmental well-being, and to discover that even subtle shifts can have lasting consequences.

ONE CITIES AND THE PATHOLOGY OF PLACE

IN 1913, the managers of the Sanitarium Association of Philadelphia shared a story about the experience of three siblings from Philadelphia at the Red Bank Sanitarium. The association's annual report recounted the tale, as told by an unnamed woman who happened to be visiting the children's neighborhood.[1]

The woman had found Mamie Donoghy sitting on the steps of a saloon with her two younger siblings, Joe and Annie. It was summertime in Philadelphia, when the temperatures could reach 90 degrees. The woman stood on the corner and, noticing Mamie, inquired, "What's your name?"

"We's de t'ree little Donoghys. My name's Mamie, I'm goin' on eight, and dat's me brother, Joe. He's goin' on seven. Dis kid's me sister Annie, she's goin' on four." Mamie chattered on, telling the stranger that a baby sister had died of whooping cough.

The woman asked Mamie where her parents were. Mamie replied that her father had died and that her mother was working, washing clothes. Like many other eldest children from urban families, Mamie was in charge during the day.

The woman likely perceived that dangers could await three young children sitting in sweltering sun on the steps of a saloon, so she invited them to go to the Red Bank Sanitarium, an open-air park across the Delaware River in Red Bank, New Jersey. The children agreed. The sanitarium was a popular place. In 1901, over 125,000 visitors used the park, with an average of almost 2,000 children and caretakers going each day.[2]

Families in the Donoghy children's neighborhood knew about the sanitarium and called out as the trio of children walked to the wharf to board the sanitarium's ferry. Mrs. McCully, a neighbor, yelled, "Don't yees get hurted or drownded, Joe Donoghy, or your mother'll beat you black and blue whin yees git back." Soon after, a group of children asked where they were going. When Mamie replied sanitarium, the children taunted, "Red Bank Bums! Red Bank Bums." Undeterred by the classist insult, the Donoghys retorted, "Sticks and stones will break our bones, but callin' names won't hurt us."

When they got to the wharf in Philadelphia, Mamie sat next to Annie and their chaperone and waited for the boat to arrive. Joe ran off to explore, returning a short time later covered in molasses and with a splinter in his foot. Finally, the ferry docked, and Mamie, Joe, and Annie boarded the vessel that shuttled them downriver to the sanitarium.

The boat sailed miles before landing at the playground's wharf. Mamie walked the gangplank to the park grounds, but before she and her siblings ran off, the woman instructed them to go "have the best time you know how." They took her words to heart. Joe went swimming, got into a skirmish with another boy, and ate two helpings of soup for lunch. Annie, the youngest, found a shady spot beneath a tree and napped the entire afternoon. Mamie joined a group of children playing tag, during which she tripped, fell into a tree, and knocked out a tooth.

At three o'clock the Donoghys boarded the steamer back to Philadelphia. As they walked through their neighborhood, Mrs. McCully, the woman who had chided the children in the morning, called, "Here's the devils back." Arriving at the saloon, the chaperone asked one last thing: "Are you glad you went, children?"

"Bet your life. Dat's the sportiest time I ever had," replied Joe. Mamie concurred, declaring, "I'm goin' to git my meother [*sic*] to take me to-morry."[3]

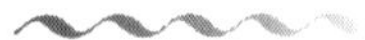

Today it seems shocking that no one objected to a stranger leading a group of children through the streets and luring them onto a boat. Neighbors admonished and jeered, but no one seemed concerned. When the managers of the Sanitarium Association of Philadelphia published this account in its 1913 annual report, they apparently assumed it would resonate with its readers. Institutions used annual reports to impress donors by highlighting success stories and good deeds. We have no way of knowing how accurate the story of the "little Donoghys" is. The association may have embellished the tale, amalgamated individuals, or even concocted the whole thing.

The story's veracity matters less than what it tells us about how people understood the interrelationship between children's bodies, health, and the urban environments where they lived and played. Impoverished children roaming the streets were a common sight, and some adults felt concerned. When looking around cities in the late nineteenth and early twentieth centuries, a growing number of professionals fretted that cities were too dirty and dangerous for the youngest inhabitants.[4]

Children ran about unsupervised, and their surroundings seemed to threaten them at every corner. Cobblestone and dirt streets were packed with horses, trolleys, and streetcars that crushed limbs and killed kids. Children played in alleys alongside stagnant water, piles of refuse, and roaming animals.[5] Over time fewer families were allowed to keep livestock in urban quarters, but packs of rabid dogs ran the streets, terrorizing children and their families.[6] Living spaces were cramped, and the outdoors did not offer much respite. Factories belched smoke, heat radiated off the streets, and the stench of refuse hung in the air.[7]

Focusing attention on cities reveals how contemporaries viewed and experienced their environments and why residents believed their surroundings debilitated children, causing disease and even death. This chapter takes us to the streets, moves into the homes of urban children and their families, and travels to sites beyond the city where working-class families sought health and reprieve. Entering these environments helps us understand why Americans believed cities were pathological places and thus sought relief in therapeutic surroundings, including the seashore. We will learn how some places, including sanatoriums, sand gardens, and seaside resorts gained cultural meaning because they were designed and experienced as sites that restored what urban centers had depleted. As we travel between the city and the spaces built to be their salubrious solutions, we learn how Americans advanced ideas about the interconnections between bodies and their surroundings.

Cities as the Cause of Disease and Death among Children

Beginning in the nineteenth century and continuing into the twentieth, a range of medical and public health professionals, social workers, and philanthropists recognized that cities were not built for children.[8] They advocated for environmental interventions to protect and restore health, while workers carved out parks, playgrounds, and rooftop classrooms. Creating healthy, green spaces was a result of concerns about infant mortality and new ideas about children's developmental needs. Beginning in the nineteenth century, child welfare advocates and psychologists claimed that children suffered from a dislocation with the natural world and saw the city as a particular threat.[9]

Nature has varied and abstract meanings, but when people discussed it in the late nineteenth century, they drew on deep-rooted, dichotomous beliefs about the city and country.[10] Nature had a pristine quality and could be found in a range of nonurban environments.[11] Healthy places included outdoor areas with fresh air, places under unobstructed skies, and medicinal waters. Such environments could be found in the vistas of farmland, pine-filled forests, the slopes of mountains, or an open expanse of beach. The built, crowded urban landscapes exemplified the opposite of all that was good and healthy.

Children also gained new cultural meaning in this era. Groups of professionals dedicated their work to understanding and promoting child development and health. They advanced arguments that childhood represented a distinct time of life that required special attention and care. This aligned with cultural shifts in children's roles within middle- and upper-class families. When more well-to-do people moved into cities, parents no longer expected children to contribute meaningfully to family economies. Children's value was increasingly sentimental, and their development needed to be nurtured by parents and professionals alike.[12]

At the same time, Americans discovered that urban children died at alarming rates. Death during childhood was not new, and parents had long mourned the death of infants and children.[13] What changed were the expectations that children should and could be healthy. But by the time reformers had identified youth as an important population to protect, American cities were too big and well established to change in large-scale ways.

These environmental constraints were new. For the first half of the nineteenth century, American cities were small and clean relative to their European counterparts, meaning healthy nature remained somewhat accessible. In 1860, New York was the largest city in the United States, with just under 814,000 residents, while Philadelphia followed with 500,000. Both were tiny compared to London's 3 million inhabitants. Over the next seventy years the United States' urban populations exploded. By 1930, New York had nearly 7 million residents, and Chicago had eclipsed Philadelphia with more than 3.3 million people, while Philadelphia's population had ballooned to nearly 2 million.[14] People flocked from the country into the cities as industries grew and jobs became concentrated in urban centers. Immigrants arrived en masse; their influx slowed only after Congress passed the Immigration Act of 1924, which established a quota system.[15] The environmental as well as the social and cultural changes alarmed many Americans and resulted in a slew of reform efforts that defined the decades around 1900.[16]

For their part, public health officials and city residents worried about epidemics. Western Europeans and their descendants in the Americas had long associated urban spaces with diseases. The bubonic plague decimated Europe's population in the 1300s, and it returned to London in the 1660s.[17] Smallpox threatened Bostonians in 1721, killing hundreds and inspiring health officials to experiment with inoculation practices.[18] Yellow fever devastated Philadelphians repeatedly in the 1790s, and it sickened residents of southern US cities throughout the nineteenth century.[19]

Epidemics' legacies, as well as new outbreaks, reinforced the idea that the more congested cities became, the more readily diseases spread. Cholera, typhoid, and diphtheria ripped through cities in the nineteenth century, killing significant portions of the population.[20] Children often suffered in great numbers. In an era before vaccines were commonplace, children lacked immunity from the range of diseases circulating, whereas many adults had survived previous exposures and were therefore less susceptible.

The extent of urban infant and child mortality made clear just how dangerous city life was for the youngest inhabitants. In the nineteenth century, Americans learned that up to 25 percent of children in the United States died before reaching twelve months of age.[21] In 1870, Philadelphia mothers gave birth to 85,957 (living) infants; that same year 19,227 children died before they turned one year old. Three years later, the Philadelphia Board of Health reported that almost 44 percent of all deaths occurred in children ten and younger.[22] New York City posted similar numbers. In 1885, New York City recorded an infant mortality rate of 247.8 per thousand. In the early twentieth century, the US Department of Commerce and Labor determined that over 30 percent of all deaths occurred in children five and younger.[23]

Statistics provided quantifiable evidence that cities harmed health. Physicians and public officials fretted not only over the number of children who died but also about the range of diseases that afflicted urban youth. In the years leading up to 1900, the Philadelphia Board of Health recorded that "cholera infantum" and other diarrheal diseases killed children, as did congestion and inflammation of lungs or brain, "debility," nutritional disorders (including marasmus and inanition), convulsions, dropsy (swelling) of the head, and cyanosis. After the turn of the century, disease categories sounded more like twenty-first-century diagnoses, including pneumonia, acute bronchitis, hydrocephalus, and congenital malformations of the heart, but broad categories such as diarrhea, debility, and other "diseases of early infancy" remained.[24] As practitioners used laboratory tests to provide specific diagnoses, nosology, the branch of medical science that focuses on the classification of disease, followed suit. This enabled practitioners and statisticians to record narrower disease categories as the cause of death.[25]

Despite diagnostic tools becoming more specific at the time, targeted treatments remained elusive. Scores of children died from gastrointestinal ailments, diphtheria, whooping cough, and various other infectious diseases, while many more suffered from chronic and debilitating conditions. Tuberculosis and rickets were especially common.[26] Although many people then and now think of tuberculosis (TB) as a disease of the lungs, when children contracted TB, it often settled into their bones, spines ("Pott's disease"), joints, and glands ("scrofula"). These forms of tuberculosis result in limbs locked in awkward angles, bent backs, and twisted spines. Open abscesses, called "sinuses," further exacerbated crippling tubercular disease in children. In the nineteenth and early twentieth centuries, physicians bemoaned such infection, as these weeping, TB-infected wounds were notoriously difficult to treat, even within newly established children's hospitals.

Rickets exemplified pediatric illnesses induced by urban conditions. In the 1890s, physician Theobald Palm published an article in *Practitioner* in which he mapped rates of rickets around the world. He found startlingly high rates within cities and lower rates in rural areas and in countries with abundant sunlight. Palm concluded that "the prevalence of rickets is as a rule in direct proportion to the massing together of the population. There are only eleven towns of over 30,000 inhabitants in which rickets is not said to be common, and three of these are health resorts." He conceded that rickets was rare in much of the United States, because most of the population still resided in rural settings. However, American cities shared rates of rickets with other industrialized landscapes. Palm noted that "the malady is met with as commonly in Philadelphia as in the large towns of Europe."[27]

Palm concluded that city life exacerbated rickets, which he believed was a disease of "malnutrition." After parsing the impacts of sanitation, water supplies, poverty, and pure air, Palm deduced that "the most salient fact with regard to the climate of those countries which enjoy immunity from rickets is the abundant sunshine and clear sky."[28] In other words, rickets was the result of air pollution and limited sunlight within congested urban spaces. While some scientists suspected that rickets was caused by a nutritional deficiency, the fact that sunbaths effectively treated and prevented the condition further supported the disease's environmental connections.

Studies of children living in American cities confirmed these impressions. In 1899 and 1900, medical journals published articles by practitioners claiming that 80 percent of Boston's children had rickets. Other studies found that immigrant and Black children were at even higher risk, with rates approaching 90 percent.[29] A 1924 article in the *Journal of the American Medical Association* claimed that 96 percent of children previously or currently had rickets, while in 1930, Memphis city health officials recorded that nearly 50 percent of white children and 87.6 percent of Black children had the disease.[30] Medical professionals maintained that children's surroundings produced conditions that induced illnesses. These beliefs did not dissipate even as disease etiology became more specific in the late nineteenth and early twentieth centuries. In fact, as diagnostic tools became more precise, they exposed just how pervasive certain medical conditions were among urban youth.

Tuberculosis was another common malady among children. In 1882, German physician Robert Koch discovered the bacillus type of bacteria that causes tuberculosis. By the 1890s, physicians used tuberculin as a diagnostic test for tuberculosis, followed by x-rays and the Pirquet skin test in the twentieth century. At the 1908 International Congress on Tuberculosis, investigators revealed that about 33 percent of children showed signs of pulmonary tuberculosis in postmortem exams, and physicians speculated an incidence of tuberculosis at 40 to 50 percent of living children. Physicians blamed cities' cramped quarters and lack of fresh air as factors that spread the disease.[31]

In addition to having rickets and tuberculosis, large numbers of urban children suffered from debility, a condition that physicians defined as a general weakness, malaise, weight loss, or a state of being run-down.[32] Scientists could not pinpoint debility's cause using laboratory-derived diagnostic tools, and it is a disease that seems elusive given our twenty-first-century medical understandings. At the time, physicians believed that debility was a weakened state of health resulting from either excessive or insufficient stimulation. Having debility rendered children and adults more susceptible to both contracting other diseases and suffering more greatly from them. In the nineteenth century, physicians tangled with the slipperiness of defining the condition. They acknowledged that often it resulted in nonspecific symptoms that largely depended on patients' sense of health.[33] Despite debility's nebulous definition, physicians and patients widely accepted it as a meaningful health condition, one bound to urban life. In this way, it was like neurasthenia, another once prominent but now defunct medical diagnosis that physicians linked to the devitalizing forces of cities.[34]

Given these prevailing beliefs, it follows that physicians and residents blamed urban life for disease. As statisticians quantified the expansive reach of illness among pediatric populations, other professionals, including physicians, educators, psychologists, social workers, and child welfare advocates, focused their attention on children's development. Childhood, they claimed, was a distinct life stage, and children required specific conditions to grow up healthy in body and mind. Many of these professionals adhered to the child study movement, a new doctrine that promoted the necessity of play and healthy environments.[35]

Moreover, adults viewed children as canaries in an urban mine. Children's smaller bodies registered environmental influences more readily than those of adults, a fact that physicians noted.[36] Prominent physician and child welfare reformer S. Josephine Baker argued that children were "plastic material" and were "the most easily molded and most responsive material that nature can give us."[37] Children's physical malleability made them more receptive to interventions seeking to improve their health, but they also readily absorbed and reacted to negative stimuli. Looking around the city, it was clear that the urban environment was dangerous for kids. Various groups set about reshaping landscapes both within and outside the city in attempts to create environments where children could grow healthy and strong.

Devil Wagons, Dead Horses, and the Problems of Play

Over the course of the nineteenth century, local government agencies attempted to quell urban health problems through sanitation and large-scale environmental reforms, such as water delivery, sewers, and trash collection.[38] Some cities widened and paved streets to shunt debris into waterways.[39] As sanitation improved from the middle to the late nineteenth century, the disease burden lessened. Yet children continued to suffer.

Despite attempts to make the built urban environment safer, it remained problematic for children in the opening decades of the twentieth century. The streets were one culprit. Child welfare advocates recognized that kids had few places to play other than city streets, where they risked being hit or crushed by horses, carriages, trolleys, and increasingly by cars.[40] In New York City, over 550 children died and more than 15,000 sustained injuries after being hit by cars in 1914 alone. Children under fifteen years of age were especially vulnerable; almost three times as many deaths occurred due to cars as from any one disease.[41] Although poor children constituted the majority of traffic accident victims, as the twentieth century progressed, middle- and upper-class children also fell victim to the so-called devil wagons.[42] The dramatic and traumatic nature of traffic accidents outraged the public, driving some witnesses to issue vigilante justice and courts to hand down harsh indictments for the drivers.

Of course, not all traffic victims died; some suffered injuries that disfigured and disabled them. Onlookers found the prevalence of crushed limbs and disabled bodies so troubling that cities passed "ugly laws" prohibiting public displays of disabilities.[43] While some urbanites sought to remove disabled children and adults from sight, others wanted to help. One wealthy woman bequeathed money to provide wooden legs to newsboys who had had an amputation after being "run over by horse cars." Newsboys rejected the gift. As Florence Kelley, a prominent women's rights activist, explained, "A little fellow who has had the luck to lose a leg appeals thereby to this same maudlin sympathy; and he appeals much more if he has a crutch and one leg than if he has sound limbs."[44]

While these newsboys approached their lives pragmatically, Kelley and other child welfare advocates fretted about children's everyday environments.[45] A consortium of professionals and parents identified the need for children to experience open spaces to be healthy. Prominent psychologist and pedagogical expert G. Stanley Hall advocated for these ideas. Beginning in the 1880s, Hall promoted the idea that childhood was a critical phase of human development and that play was crucial to children's—especially boys'—physical, mental, and civic maturation. Hall delivered this message to popular and scientific audiences alike.[46]

Some cities had recognized the benefits of providing children with safe outdoor environments. Boston pioneered "sand gardens" in 1885.[47] Dr. Marie Zakrzewska, who founded the New England Hospital for Women and Children in 1862, imported the idea for sandboxes from Germany after seeing children frolic on sandpiles during a visit to Berlin. When Zakrzewska returned home, she partnered with the Massachusetts Emergency and Hygiene Association to construct a sand garden so that "slum children" could have a place to escape the congestion and filth of their living quarters.[48]

The first sandpiles were such a success among children and their mothers that the women leading the hygiene association sought and received permission from the city to install gigantic sandboxes in poor neighborhoods and schoolyards during the summer. A local construction firm donated the sand for summertime play.[49] The sandboxes and sandpiles caught the attention of Frederick Law Olmsted, America's premier landscape architect. He dedicated space for children's sand gardens in the Charlesbank section of the Emerald Necklace, a park system he designed to improve the health of Bostonians.[50] Other cities followed suit. In the 1890s, Jane Addams, the prominent social reformer, opened one at Hull House, the settlement home she ran in Chicago. New York joined the trend, establishing sand gardens in Hell's Kitchen and the Lower East Side. San Francisco had one by 1898.[51]

Sand gardens provided children with a safe place outdoors, removed from the gutters and streets. Women were central to promoting these spaces as environments where children could exercise their bodies and minds, free of the baleful influences of the city.[52] Famous male colleagues and wealthy families followed their lead. Sandpiles were so pervasive that G. Stanley Hall documented their benefits. In an 1897 pamphlet, Hall recounted the experience of Dr. and Mrs. A, who installed a sandpile at their summer cottage. As Hall explained, Mrs. A "persisted, not without some inconvenience, in having a load of fine clean sand hauled from a distant beach and dumped in the yard for the children to play in."[53]

Sand gardens were a precursor to playgrounds. In the early twentieth century, a playground movement gained steam in the United States, and organizers promoted these spaces as a vehicle to teach children "how best to use their leisure."[54] Expanding on the original sandbox design, new playgrounds incorporated additional structures. Adults, including police officers, orchestrated activities, much to many children's dismay.[55]

Playgrounds carved out some small spaces for children within the city, but child welfare advocates were unsatisfied. Children, they argued, needed access to larger swaths of land. By the early twentieth century they had diagnosed this as a problem with urban design. At the 1911 Child Welfare Exhibit in Chicago, Charles Zueblin, editor of *Twentieth Century Magazine*, lamented that "we do not have to go very far back to find the time that neither the houses nor the streets nor the parks were planned with any recognition of the children."[56] Tapping into the latest psychological theories, including race betterment ideologies, Zueblin argued that cities' lack of open space prevented children from attaining their fullest physical and mental potentials.[57] Urban parks, he noted, were a recent phenomenon, and he complained that they were meant "to be enjoyed only by those who were in advancing years" and "that children should be permitted simply to visit the parks."[58]

The lack of access was troubling because landscape architects designed parks to improve the health of the city and its inhabitants. For instance, Olmsted viewed Central Park in New York City as the "lungs" of the city, providing reservoirs of fresh air that could invigorate urban masses. His Emerald Necklace park system in Boston was a hygienic intervention, redressing declining environmental and human health through ponds and playgrounds.[59]

But Zueblin expressed his irritation that too many residents, including children, had difficulty accessing healthy urban landscapes likes those Olmsted designed. He denounced Philadelphia as emblematic of the problem. Philadelphia boasted an expansive park system, yet Zueblin criticized its remote location, which meant that "a great majority of the inhabitants never used it because they never discovered its location and never knew about it."[60] He also expressed his frustration that cities restricted use of beaches; one such city was Boston, which prohibited residents from using them for bathing until 1866. Zueblin even admonished the conference's host city of Chicago because it permitted bathing in "only three little places on the twenty-seven miles of lake frontage."[61]

As noted above, children could access some small spaces in the city, Zueblin explained that such places, including playgrounds, were important because "there is the training of these children in more than mere play, and in that you will see a necessity for the democracy of the future; you will see in the wise use of leisure a contribution to the whole growth of democracy that will appear in the very fibre of the history-makers of the future." He asked his audience, "How shall we teach them to use their leisure?"[62]

Reformers advocated for playgrounds, identifying them as being beneficial to children's physical and moral development.[63] Educator and author T. Benjamin Atkins linked play with health. He told his readers (whom he modestly defined as "all those who were once children themselves") that "every healthful child is a playful child."[64] He explained, "When the child plays it is for the creation of human life. When the muscles play it is for the creation of physical life. When the mind plays it is for the creation of mental life. It is through play that nature develops the child in all the faculties, both physical and mental."[65]

Atkins tied urban children's inability to play to their poor health. He wrote, "Play is necessary to health. The fearful mortality among children in crowded flats and tenement houses where the play-grounds are restricted does more to reduce the average of human life than any other cause, intemperance excepted."[66] Atkins recommended that his readers visit a surgical sanitarium as proof. He told people they would witness "hundreds of different forms of deformity, withered limbs hanging hideous and helpless not half their natural size; crooked spines, dwarfed bodies, men's heads on bodies not larger than those of children."[67] The reason, according to Atkins? "The defective limb had by some accident been disqualified for free play." The remedy was straightforward: "Remove the impediment. Give the dwarfed limb its natural activity and nature will do the rest, restore it whole like the other."[68]

While Atkins did not delineate specific diseases, his references to "withered limbs" and "crooked spines" invoked images of children suffering from rickets and tuberculosis. If movement and play restored mobility, they could also prevent children from becoming ill in the first place. Atkins alluded to this idea when he referenced the "fearful mortality" among urban poor, the very same populations plagued by disabling and debilitating conditions.

Yet for decades children could not easily access parks within the city. Ever creative, children embraced the spaces they had. Some jumped rope or played jacks or hopscotch on sidewalks.[69] Dead horses also captured children's attention; youngsters used carcasses to play king of the hill or ran and jumped on the horses' bodies, knowing the animal's bladder might burst and release a horrid-smelling wave.[70] Other kids swam in rivers, apparently ignoring restrictions, and would have to dodge feces when and where the sewer pipes discharged. In the streets children invented various ball games, in defiance of motorists and police. Florence Kelley noted with frustration that New York City officers arrested eight thousand boys in one year for "playing ball—that was the charge against them in court."[71]

While parks may have helped remove children from the dangers of city streets, there were not enough playgrounds to serve them all. Moreover, playgrounds were still urban institutions. Children could run and build muscles in these parks, which was better than remaining in cramped indoor environments or playing in dangerous streets, but people complained about the smoke and soot that darkened the skies.[72] In 1919, authors in Chicago lamented that "there is no sky now," while a Milwaukee resident detailed the inescapable and visceral experience of pollution, writing, "I swallow it. It fills my eyes, chocks [*sic*] my bronchial tubes. It comes between me and the sun and I see my fellow beings suffer day by day."[73] In Pittsburgh the pollution was so severe that streetlights remained on during the day so that residents could navigate the urban terrain.[74]

Sandpiles, playgrounds, and parks afforded some children a safer alternative to the city street, but these urban spaces could not provide access to fresh air or sunshine. Recognizing that cities' outdoor environments remained injurious, early twentieth-century child welfare workers set their sights on the private spaces of families' homes to protect children from urban ills.

Healthy Homes?

Well into the twentieth century, most health care took place within the home. Mothers' caregiving roles included creating and maintaining healthy houses as a form of protecting children from dirt and disease.[75] This was no easy task. Upper- and middle-class urban mothers planted flower boxes with blooms that "sweetened" and purified the air, they hung deodorizing sachets in closets, and they swept, cleaned, and chased out dirt and vermin.[76] New technologies emerged to "help" women clean and improve domestic sanitation. While women embraced some devices, such as washing machines, many other tools created new cultural expectations of cleanliness and increased the hours mothers and other women spent doing housework.[77]

In addition to keeping their homes free from dirt and germs, upper- and middle-class mothers oversaw the installation of indoor plumbing in their homes. They ensured that the plumbing system worked properly so sewer gas did not seep into the house.[78] Working-class mothers did not need to attend to such issues, however; their homes often lacked plumbing and electricity.

Mothers' health and caregiving responsibilities were never easy, but working-class women bore seemingly insurmountable barriers to keeping healthy homes. Many of their residences lacked proper ventilation, had poor drainage and little sunlight, and were often crowded with people and animals. Moreover, families often rented their living spaces, which further limited their ability to effect changes. Domestic environments were microcosms of the problems outside their doors, and child welfare advocates identified urban homes as additional pathological places within the city.

When social workers made home visits, they recognized the problem. In December 1921, a social worker for the pediatric unit at the Hospital of the University of Pennsylvania ("Penn") readied herself for a home visit. She would be seeing a former patient named Nick who had received treatment for "a bad burn." As the social worker prepared to visit his neighborhood, where many Italian immigrants lived, she conjured a romantic vision. She expected to visit "a broad paved street with double trolley lines, new, two-story houses and small Italian stores." Yet, as she neared the patient's house, the "paved street terminated and beyond was a region of dirt roads, corn fields, dumps and old tumbled down planter houses."[79]

The social worker searched for Nick's house. Asking the corner druggist for directions, she learned the family lived "in a 'shack house' at the end of a muddy lane, mostly fenced by rusty bed springs." Nick's house was "a two-room hovel standing by itself in a field, there is no under-drainage." She lamented that "there were two dogs, a cat, and a baby in the hot dirty cluttered up kitchen."[80] The home's poor physical conditions were compounded by the family's financial circumstances. Nick's father was unemployed, and the family owed the grocer $100. To make matters worse, two boys needed medical treatment. Nick's mother did not speak English and reported she was unable to make it to the hospital by herself.

Attempting to help, the worker approached the family's priest, who replied that he could not help Nick's family because he had hundreds of others living in similar conditions. He chided her, saying that he was "a busy man and had no time for 'sociability.'" The worker arranged for the local housing association to investigate the home and had the social service department refer the family to the Italian Federation for financial assistance and employment for the father. The worker concluded that she would "try to persuade the parents to let Nick go to the Country."[81]

When the social worker entered Nick's home, she saw many of the same problems that defined the urban outdoors. Both environments were dirty, crowded, and lacked fresh air. Far from offering protection, working-class children's housing seemed to exacerbate poor health. Social workers, nurses, and medical professionals expressed their concerns, and some criticized parents' caregiving ability. In January 1919, Helen Lois Jones, one of the home visitors who represented Penn hospital pediatric wards, recorded her experience with Lucy, a young girl with influenza. She wrote that "though an Italian [Lucy] has beautiful bronze hair and blue eyes." In contrast, Jones characterized Lucy's sister Concetta as "a typical undernourished Italian baby," who was fed a diet of "buttermilk and macaroni." Jones deemed that Lucy, however, was healthy and ate properly.[82] Jones concluded that the family's care of baby Concetta was problematic likely because it conflicted with American medical professionals' advice regarding infant feeding practices. Jones condemned Concetta's care as being typical of Italian families.

Some social workers freely expressed their bias and judged families, but others exhibited compassion, praising mothers' willingness to work with their children's health providers.[83] One social worker recorded that her patient, Paul, came from a "nice Italian family." She was impressed by Paul's mother, who spoke English well, seemed "quite intelligent," and kept her home very clean. The worker determined that Paul's poor health was a result of his mother's practices of only opening the windows at night during warm weather and giving her son a bath just once a week in the winter. The social worker instructed the mother to give Paul "cool sponges and plenty of fresh air." Leaving the family's home, she felt confident that Paul's mother would follow her directions.[84]

Many social workers and nurses partnered with mothers to reform the home environment and the child-care practices within it. Their willingness to collaborate to create healthier homes even extended to mothers who were unable to fully comply with accepted standards of child rearing, such as keeping a sick child away from siblings. Moments of alignment are important because they show that provider-patient interactions could be mutual and collaborative, not just top-down, heavy-handed, and unfairly judgmental.[85]

While some families adopted the practices that professionals preached, others ignored advice or believed that adjusting the home was not enough. In March 1922, the Babies' Hospital in Philadelphia contacted the Penn hospital's social services department to "warn" them about the Presti family. The Babies' Hospital had discharged their child, but the baby was unhealthy, weighing just thirteen pounds despite being a year old. Sure enough, only four days after being discharged from the Babies' Hospital, the infant was admitted to the Penn hospital. The father arrived at the social services department "weeping" and requesting to be sent to the country. The social worker noted that the "home conditions are at the back of his and the baby's poor health," although they did not identify specific problems.[86] This father's request suggests he saw his home life as the root of his health problems and the country as a healthful solution.

Working-class families knew they could only do so much to create healthier urban homes. Small modifications such as opening windows or giving children baths more frequently might be possible. But they could not afford to alter their homes to improve drainage, renovate for better ventilation, or move into larger homes that could more comfortably fit their families.

Environmental interventions were difficult, regardless of the scale or site. Family and child welfare advocates recommended urban dwellers go to the country, where it was cooler, cleaner, and the sun remained unencumbered by pollution. Nonurban environments were less populated, and fewer people meant more space, more fresh air, and less exposure to disease. In the country mothers did not have to battle urban dirt, grime, and refuse.

While the scope and scale of environmental interventions shifted over time, they did not dislodge the pervasive sentiment that the spaces where children lived and played determined their health and well-being. The city remained a pathological place, and physicians, families, and child welfare advocates continued to look beyond the city for salubrious solutions.

Escaping the City to Search for Health

Urban residents were not environmentally myopic; they could see that fleeing to the country was a healthy solution to treat and prevent disease. Wealthier families took vacations or summered at country homes to escape the heat and its corresponding epidemics. Some looked to the mountains, with their promise of pine trees that purified the air. Regions like the Adirondacks and White Mountains attracted hay fever sufferers, promising relief from allergy-like symptoms.[87] Physicians established sanitariums for tuberculosis sufferers and bathhouses at hot springs to care for sick and run-down patients. Historians have examined how tourists sought refreshment on mountaintops and at spas, detailing the range of ways Americans have imagined them as sites of health and well-being.[88]

Working-class families also participated in these migrations, albeit on a different scale. Some took excursions to nearby shores, creating accessible leisure corridors. By the nineteenth century, charitable groups were providing working-class children with time spent away from the city, at least temporarily. The Fresh Air Fund in New York City and the Children's Country Week Association in Philadelphia sent children outside the city for days or weeks. During the school year some districts built outdoor spaces for class instruction. Mothers and children in Boston and New York took advantage of their cities' floating hospitals. These hospital ships shuttled mothers and children for daily rides in the city's bays and promoted "fresh air as medicine."[89] These organizations shared a foundational belief that urban families, and children in particular, needed to escape the noxious exhalations and vitiated air—the ambient atmosphere rendered dangerous by human respiration.[90]

Philanthropic groups promoted this environmental ideology, as well as their programs' benefits, while soliciting financial support. In the early twentieth century, the New York Association for Improving the Condition of the Poor published an appeal entitled "From Stifling Tenement to Seashore and Country" and highlighted the need for urban children to leave the city. R. Fulton Cutting, president of the association, queried his readers: "Do you know that the New Yorker living below Fourteenth Street has an average of only 18 square feet of breathing space? Can you imagine anyone more in need of fresh air outings than these dwellers in sultry homes, hemmed in by scorching pavements?" Yet fresh air, readers learned, was unattainable if these folks remained in the city, as "fresh breezes and outdoor freedom are made impossible by congestion." The advertisement implored readers to help "mothers, children, and babies broke with toil, ill-nurtured, or frail" by supporting trips to "the country or at Sea Breeze, our seashore Home at Coney Island." There impoverished families could access "a bit of sunshine" and "pure air."[91] Photographs surrounded the text of the plea. They provided visual evidence of the urban burdens that children endured and the pleasures that awaited at the beach. Along the left side of the circular, wan children, some carrying heavy loads, roam city streets. The images are a stark contrast to the photographs that frame the right side of the text. Scanning those pictures, viewers saw children grinning in the sun, bare feet dangling in the water, and hair tousled by the sea breezes. A photograph labeled "The Bathing Hour at Sea Breeze" lines the header. The white foam of a gentle wave encircles the legs of dozens of bathers who wade into the sea, while children play in the sand. The photographs offer visual evidence of the association's claims that donations enable women and children to regain health, cheer, and a "new start for the next [school] year" by accessing the fresh air outside of the city.[92]

Philadelphians sought similar sites of respite. The Sanitarium Association of Philadelphia, where Mamie Donoghy and her siblings went, ferried children and their caretakers from Philadelphia to the playground down the river during summer weekdays. The association's work illustrates how private residents, the state, physicians, and families invested in environmental interventions to tackle urban problems. Looking at how child welfare advocates structured solutions tells us how people defined urban landscapes as health problems and the ways they conceptualized the risk of not intervening. The sanitarium's built environment reflected the cultural and medical ideologies that children needed green surroundings to grow into healthy future citizens.

In general, sanitariums, like other rural health care institutions, served people who were suffering from chronic conditions or were convalescing from acute illness. The institutions were often located in the pastoral landscapes or mountains and thus provided patients access to fresh air. Both the buildings and grounds proffered health. The Sanitarium Association of Philadelphia conformed to some of these trends. It admitted children and mothers without specified medical problems.

The association first opened in 1877 on Windmill Island, a dot of land in the Delaware River. The organizers chose the island, nestled between the cities of Philadelphia, Pennsylvania, and Camden, New Jersey, because "even in the hottest season, a fresh, pure, and invigorating air prevails." They celebrated the island's "abundant shade, a beautiful lawn, and such simple accessories of childhood's enjoyments as swings, hammocks, and baby-coaches."[93]

The managers exulted in the island's proximity to two major cities because it made for convenient day trips. But Windmill Island's location also led to its deterioration. The ports of Philadelphia and Camden were busy, and the island was an inconvenient obstacle to shipping lanes between Pennsylvania and New Jersey. Tides, along with poor drainage, further threatened the island. Its death knell rang when a tornado struck the island and uprooted many of its trees, which were then washed away.[94] The association's board decided to move the institution downriver, selecting a largely undeveloped site in Red Bank, New Jersey.

The managers celebrated the new, more remote location as being environmentally advantageous. It benefited from the "westerly or prevailing summer winds sweeping around the curve of the Delaware at this point," as well as its "perfect drainage for all waste matters; freedom from malaria, and the pollution of the surrounding waters from the sewage of a great city."[95] The managers encouraged potential benefactors to visit Red Bank to witness the improvement in children's health and happiness. The institution promised sights of

> multitudes of little ones, gathered from the slums and by-ways of the great city, enjoying the novelty of a ride upon the river, exhilarated by the fresh, pure breezes from off the water; to notice the almost magic effect of a change of air upon the sick infants removed from the fever-laden atmosphere of crowded and unhealthy homes; to observe the mirth and healthful amusement of the thousands of children gathered together upon the spacious grounds of the park, and the comfort and tender care of the sick ones amply provided for under shady trees in the fresh air and in the well-ventilated wards of the hospital building.[96]

It is not clear how many prospective donors heeded this call, but working-class children and mothers arrived in droves. In 1883, H. F. Keyser, one of the sanitarium's officers, compiled statistics on the number of infants, children, and adults who used the sanitarium each day. On May 31, only seventy-six people came. By July 23, over fourteen hundred women and children had visited on a single day. The numbers fluctuated over the season, which the managers attributed to the weather. Keyser also recorded the weather in a daily admissions table, noting if it was clear, cloudy, or raining. Even on rainy days, however, hundreds of families took advantage of the park.[97]

The sanitarium also reported air temperatures, to establish its environmental superiority over the city. For seventy-eight days in 1883, the institution recorded the temperatures at 9:00 a.m., noon, 3:00 p.m., and 6:00 p.m. and contrasted them to recordings taken at an optician's office located at 628 Chestnut Street in Philadelphia. The variance was often stark. The sanitarium registered numbers in the 70s or 80s and had more days in the 60s than in the 90s. The city could be five to six degrees warmer than the sanitarium, and on some days the differential was even greater. The sanitarium's cooler temperatures beckoned children and mothers and provided quantitative proof of the institution's beneficial environment.[98]

Weather charts confirmed what physicians and parents already knew: cities' heat endangered children, and time in the country provided relief. Managers published a table of the mortality rate for Philadelphia children under the age of five. Since the sanitarium's opening in 1877, the infant mortality rate in Philadelphia had steadily declined. In 1872, young children represented nearly 44 percent of the total deaths in the city; ten years later that figure had fallen to just over 36 percent. The writers acknowledged that the correlation may have been coincidental but pleaded, "May we not be justified in concluding, that the Sanitarium and the Children's Country Week and kindred institutions have been, in some degree, instrumental in lessening the death-rate as above noted? Assuredly some such result should follow the extended efforts of these beneficent organizations!"[99]

The report reminded readers that "the intense heat, unhealthy surroundings, and circumstances attending poverty" sapped children's health.[100] The sanitarium provided an environmental tonic to city life by giving children "fresh air, by the supply of wholesome food, facilities for bathing and cleanliness, clothing to the destitute, proper attention for the sick and last, but not least, by the benefit of instruction in hygiene and the care of children."[101]

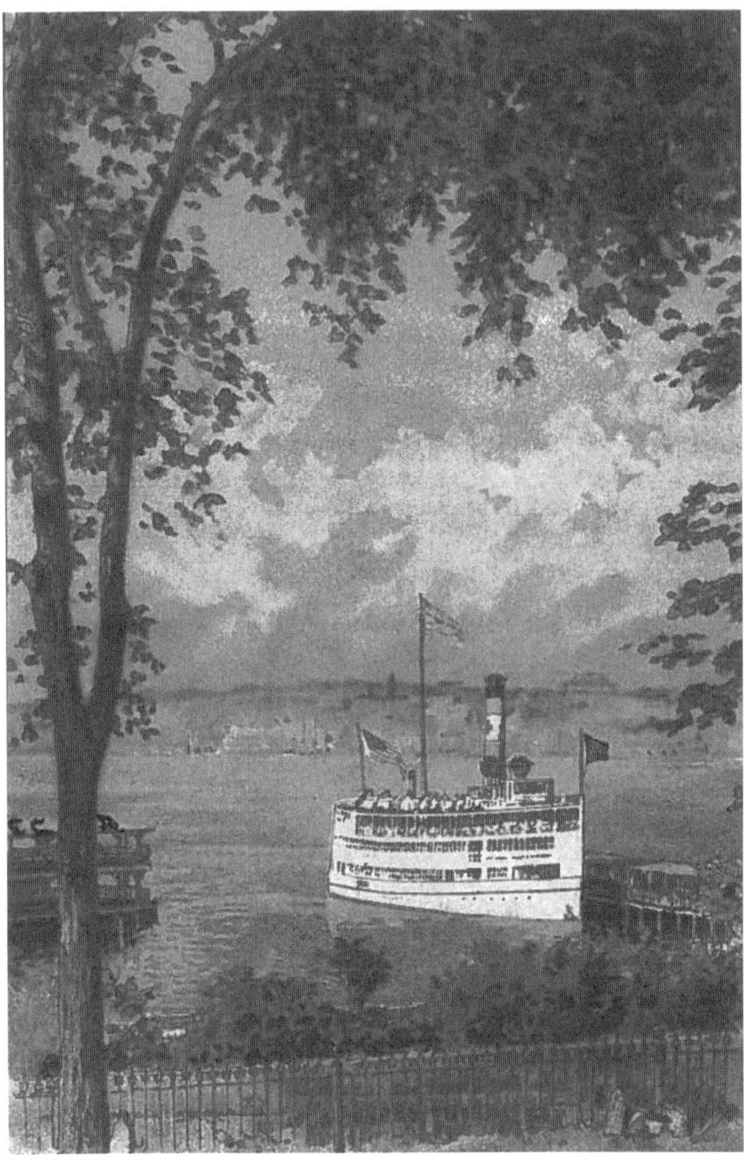

FIGURE 2. "The Boston Floating Hospital at Her Pier at North End Park, As Seen from Copp's Hill." Postcard with drawing of the Boston Floating Hospital on the front. The reverse side notes that the hospital provides free treatment "with the benefit of sea air for hundreds of sick babies and little children during the heat of summer." Author's collection.

Fresh air was medicine, and the sanitarium dispensed it to thousands every summer.[102]

Philadelphia families and child welfare advocates were not alone in seeking environmental solutions to improve children's health outside of cities. Boston-based Reverend Rufus B. Tobey encountered "crowds of children and mothers with infants in arms walking up and down the South Boston bridge" every evening as he traveled home from work. The mothers were seeking a wisp of fresh air or a cool breeze to bring relief to their babies.[103] Tobey was inspired to help and established the Boston Floating Hospital, a barge that brought mothers and their children on daily rides around Boston Bay. On board the ship, women and infants basked in the cool, salty breezes they could not access on city streets. Like the Sanitarium Association of Philadelphia, the Boston Floating Hospital reported positive, even life-saving outcomes after a day outside the city. Boston's mothers supported the hospital by seeking admission for their babies.

Mothers and children in New York City did the same. As in Boston, mothers clamored for admission to fresh air institutions. Women lauded these temporary escapes, at least according to journalists. In 1909, reporter Lewis Edwin Theiss published an article detailing New York City's fresh air work in *Outing Magazine*. He told readers of amazing transformations of "fading children freshened into new life, of dying mothers snatched from the grave, of despairing families heartened anew for the battle of life."[104] Theiss highlighted New York City's Fresh Air Fund, Edgewater Crèche, the Children's Aid Society health homes at Coney Island and Bath Beach, Sea Breeze Hospital, and the St. John's Guild floating and seaside hospitals.

Theiss reported that mothers pursued admission to these fresh air and seaside institutions. In New York, one mother made her way to the pier where the floating hospital was docked. She carried a "fading infant in her arms." Arriving at the hospital, she proclaimed (in Theiss's recounting) that "Bambino verra verra sick but the biga ship maka well."[105] Taken at face value, the pejorative reporting notwithstanding, this mother believed that getting out of the city and into fresh air would benefit her child. The notion that working-class families sought and advocated for access to healthier, nonurban environments is supported by other institutions' records, including the

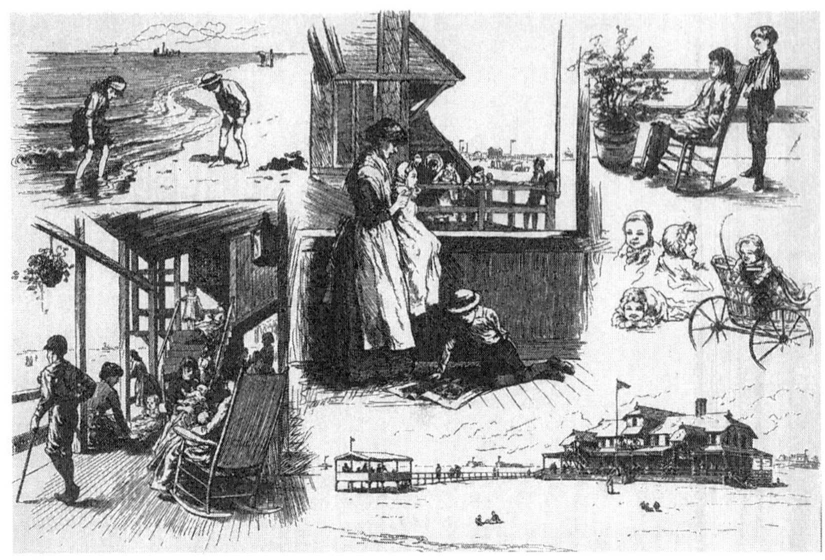

FIGURE 3. "The Children's Health Home at Coney Island." Series of sketches of children playing at the beach, many of them sick or with a physical disability, some with their mothers. *Harper's Young People*, August 26, 1884, 681. Author's collection.

Philadelphia-based hospital social worker who recorded Mr. Presti's request to be sent to the country to rehabilitate.

Children also understood that cities depleted their health, and they too requested time in the countryside to restore their well-being. One girl wrote to a fresh air program in New York requesting "to get my brother and sisters to the country as soon as you can, for we are almost dying with the heat." She wished to go too, writing, "I can work and make myself useful. But if you ain't got no room, for me, send my brother and sisters."[106] This girl's appeal was not youthful hyperbole. She likely saw her younger siblings' languishing health, and she sought to remedy the problem the best way she knew: by getting them into the cooler countryside.

Another child reminisced about her experience at a fresh air institution in Nyack, New York. The girl, who lived in one of New York City's tenements, reported to her teacher, "It was just as nice as I dreamed it was, and I ain't never going to wake up."[107] She ostensibly compared her happy, ethereal experience in the country to the hard realities of living in the hot and crowded city during the summer months.

Institutions that gave children and families access to nonurban environments remained popular well into the twentieth century, despite massive shifts in medical knowledge, sanitation, and public health practices. In fact, the popularity of institutions such as the Sanitarium Association of Philadelphia and Boston Floating Hospital soared in the late nineteenth and early twentieth centuries. Americans maintained a deep conviction that cities were pathological places and sought spaces of health beyond urban boundaries.

CONCERNS ABOUT CITIES' IMPACT on health were not new in the late nineteenth and early twentieth century, nor were the environmental interventions to ameliorate those effects.[108] One change was the focus on children. Reformers emphasized the interconnection between urban children's health and the environments where they lived and played.

Adults' interests in maintaining children's health resulted in new spaces in cities and increased attention to children's surroundings. But even the most ardent advocates for urban environmental reforms acknowledged that their interventions could not replicate the experience of the countryside or the beach. As early as 1889, Ellen M. Towner, chairwoman for the Committee of Playgrounds with the Massachusetts Emergency and Hygiene Association, conceded "that the joys of our playgrounds rival those of green fields, or that our sand-heaps are a fitting substitute for the wide sea-beach, we do not claim."[109] Play in the city could not approximate being in more salubrious environments like the seashore.

As more people moved to urban centers, children continued to contract and die from infectious diseases, fight for space to play on streets and sidewalks, and suffer from the range of ailments that debilitated the nation's youth. Leaving the city remained a logical remedy, given these realities. While some city dwellers continued to travel to the mountains for relief, urban Americans increasingly looked to their coasts. Many of the northeastern cities of the United States were located near the Atlantic Ocean. The sea breezes that bathed visitors ensured that the air never became vitiated or stagnant. Sunlight along the coast was plentiful and amplified by the ocean; taking a dip in the sea promised a respite from sweltering summer days.

Physicians lauded the health benefits accrued from a sojourn to the sea and wrote prescriptions to travel there. Prospectors staked money on developing America's eastern seashore into a series of health resorts. Railroad companies laid tracks between cities and the shore, providing access to an increased number of visitors. Philanthropists built hospitals. In the end, patients eagerly consumed their marine medication, and tourists followed.

As the twentieth century dawned, more and more trains whisked urban families between the city and the shore, for a day, a week, or the summer. Knowledge of the beaches' rejuvenating properties grew. Physicians, nurses, and social workers applauded patients' health and healing at the coast. They produced and disseminated scientific and medical evidence of the marine environment's therapeutic benefits. Tourists, working-class mothers, and children availed themselves of a trip to the beach. As they traveled between the city and the shore, they reinforced cultural and medical beliefs that the beach was an antidote to urban life.

TWO FINDING CURES AT THE SHORE

PICTURE THE BEACH. Perhaps you conjured an expanse of sand, visible between bodies of various ages, shapes, and sizes. Colorful umbrellas shield some people, while sunbathers lie languidly beneath the sun. Children scatter, chasing waves, digging in the sand, and throwing balls. Bathers bob in the ocean, while surfers ride the waves, and a swimmer methodically moves parallel to the shore. You might picture a beachgoer's hair tousled by the breeze or even imagine the smell of salt-laden air as you take a deep breath. You hear waves crashing, gulls squawking, and the tinny song of ice cream trucks.

Before the mid-nineteenth century, most Americans could not conjure such images. Until that time, the nation's shores were largely empty spaces. Few non–Native Americans made the beach their home. For centuries Europeans and their American descendants feared the sea: it swelled, stormed, and harbored beasts.[1] Sailors lost their lives on the ocean. Immigrants, both voluntary and forced, knew the dangers, discomforts, and potential for death during ocean passage.[2] Of course some people lived near the ocean. Fishing and whaling villages dotted the salty edges of the land. But the seashore did not exist as the popular tourist site we know today.

The beach emerged as travel destination in Europe in the eighteenth century, when members of royal and elite society began to sojourn at the seaside. They saw the shore as an environment with the potential to heal and to restore energy.[3] Wealthy Americans followed suit in the nineteenth century. In the early to mid-1800s, they built luxurious accommodations so as to escape pestilential cities and plantations, traveling to places such as Cape May, New Jersey, and Newport, Rhode Island.[4] Gradually, more Americans sought time at the seashore, as a site that would rejuvenate the health that cities had depleted.

The practice of traveling for health was not novel. Doctors had long advised that changing one's environment could improve health. Physicians studied and analyzed environments for their potential to either cause or cure disease. Mountains provided a place of relief as well, particularly for folks suffering from hay fever or tuberculosis.[5] Doctors celebrated the fresh, pine-scented air as particularly healing. Medicinal springs and spas flourished, as did mountaintop escapes. Physicians in the United States and Europe supported the enterprise by sending patients for water cures, which entailed bathing, drinking, and being blasted by spring-fed showers in attempts to restore health.[6]

Doctors also prescribed sea voyages. Despite the arduous conditions and limited food supplies, physicians advocated ocean travel for debilitated men.[7] The prevailing medical wisdom was that the bracing sea air and undulations of the ship fortified travelers' health. Few people could afford such a voyage, however. The time away from employment and family limited sea voyaging to wealthy men. By the mid-nineteenth century, though, doctors had recognized that the seashore could serve a similar function for an even wider range of patients. The beach offered many practical advantages to ocean travel; it was closer to home, less expensive, and accessible to men, women, and children.

This chapter situates the seashore alongside other therapeutic landscapes. It explores how physicians helped establish Americans' vision of the beach as a destination that restored health and strength. It also shows that medical professionals heralded the beach as particularly efficacious for families and children from all social classes. Doctors wrote lengthy books, published scores of professional articles and popular testimonies, held conferences exalting the health benefits of the seashore, and staffed institutions to provide urban youth with "marine medication."[8] Physicians' dedication to seashore therapies reinforced medical ideologies that elevated environmental cures and health care for over seven decades. Their practices maintained that sea air, seawater, and sunbathing were curative and preventative interventions.

We will also learn how physicians and scientists explained the seashore's therapeutic effects through scientific investigations and how this approach gradually eroded an ability to see the seashore as a holistically healthful landscape. When doctors first started sending patients to the beach in the mid-nineteenth century, they pointed to patients' transformed bodies as physical proof of efficacy: children who left cities sick, scrawny, and weak returned from the seashore healthy, ruddy cheeked, and robust. With the rise of laboratory-based scientific medicine in the late nineteenth and early twentieth centuries, even dramatic corporal changes were no longer enough. Physicians applied laboratory methods to study the seashore's curative mechanisms and isolated specific chemicals and pathways that improved health.[9]

As their therapeutic vision narrowed, physicians distilled the seashore and its healthy components. They celebrated saline but not the ocean, UV rays rather than the sun, and ozone but not the sea breezes. Physicians may have become more myopic, but they never rejected claims that time at the seashore could cure disease and restore health. However, their approach to determining marine medication's efficacy had lasting impacts. By the 1930s, the beach was still being seen as beneficial but no longer as a holistic landscape of health and healing.

The Spectacle of Children's Health

Beginning in the mid-nineteenth century and continuing into the twentieth century, seashore hospitals admitted pediatric patients and highlighted a medical faith in the coast as a site of healing. The first seaside hospital opened in 1856 in Viareggio, a city along Italy's northwestern seaboard. Four years later France opened Berck-sur-Mer to care for Parisian children who suffered from urban maladies such as tuberculosis. Similar institutions sprang up along the seaboards near major urban centers in Europe and the northeastern United States, as well as outside of Buenos Aires, Argentina. By 1914, more than eighty seashore hospitals across three continents had admitted patients.[10] While seaside hospitals reflected their regional and national contexts, the similarities among such institutions outweighed minor differences. Across these hospitals physicians employed marine medication, a treatment program that consisted of sea air, seawater, and eventually sunbathing.

They also often admitted pediatric patients, a practice that aligned with a burgeoning interest in children's health care. In the United States pediatric hospitals began serving urban children in the mid- to late nineteenth century.[11] Many of these were small institutions, operating out of converted homes in the nation's largest cities. While physicians treated children, only a handful dedicated their entire practice to children's health care at the turn of the twentieth century. Pediatrics became professionally formalized in 1930, when a group of physicians split with the American Medical Association and formed the American Academy of Pediatrics.[12]

Although the profession of pediatrics was nascent, parents and practitioners went to incredible lengths to access health care for children. Three stories, all involving children and the ocean, highlight this reality. The first occurred in the early morning hours of December 2, 1885, in Newark, New Jersey. A rabid dog terrorized the city, biting six children and seven dogs. Rabies was not the most common disease that killed children, but people knew its terrifying effects. Those who contracted it suffered a range of issues that progressed over weeks. Symptoms could start mildly as the initial wound healed. Victims might feel weak or uncomfortable, as if they had the flu. As the disease progressed, patients would experience intense muscle spasms, hallucinations, and insomnia. They developed hydrophobia, a fear of drinking water.[13] Newspaper reporters would relay horrific stories, including one of a child with rabies whose screams could be heard a block away. The *New York Times* published an account of one young victim who thrashed so violently that three grown men had to hold him down.[14]

When news spread about the "Newark Boys," the public understood that the children were in mortal danger. Fortunately, French physician Louis Pasteur had recently developed a treatment for rabies, and a local Newark physician became determined to raise funds to send the children to Paris for the cure. He published a plea, and people quickly answered the doctor's appeal. Pasteur agreed to treat the children, and on December 10, 1885, the four boys boarded a steamer bound for Paris.[15]

Across the United States newspapers regaled readers with accounts of the boys' experiences as they made their way across the Atlantic Ocean to be cured by one of the most famous practitioners at the time. An article relayed that one of the boys exclaimed that the rabies shot tickled and felt "like the bite of a big mosquito."[16] Another report described the boys' triumphant return, describing the children as exemplars of health with "rosy cheeks and sparkling eyes and happy as the day is long."[17] The boys arrived home to great fanfare.

People paid money to see the boys in person, to witness what seemed like a medical miracle. The excitement at the boys' recovery reflected popular interest in medical advances and a desire to witness results firsthand.

"Baby incubator" shows, the second story, support the conclusion that children's health gained spectacular traction into the early twentieth century. On the boardwalks of Coney Island, New York, barkers yelled, "Don't pass the babies by!" If their curiosity was piqued, visitors could enter an ornate brick building with large block letters that announced, "INFANT INCUBATORS." The exhibit's portico featured the message "Infant Incubators with Living Infants." After shelling out twenty-five cents, tourists walked around a room where they peered at tiny live babies nestled in machines that regulated temperature, much like chicken egg incubators. The visitors saw nurses attending to the infants' needs, with Dr. Martin Couney overseeing the operation.

Although some medical professionals decried Couney as a quack and dismissed his operation as a sideshow, these babies had no other medical options. When Couney opened his baby display in 1903, premature infants' parents were equipped with little more than a wish and a prayer. Only a few hospitals had nurseries, and the first neonatal unit to care for sick and preterm infants did not open in the United States until 1960. While incubator babies' survival rate may not have reached the 100 percent that Couney claimed, it did approach 85 percent, an astonishing success rate given that even healthy babies often succumbed to disease.

Couney's baby display was not the only one of its kind. Atlantic City boasted its own incubator show, and similar exhibits appeared at world's fairs and expositions. Even Americans who could not see them firsthand could read about them in newspaper stories that detailed the experiments. The shows' cultural popularity inculcated a belief that medical technologies saved the lives of even the weakest and most vulnerable patients.[18] They also reminded viewers that infants' immediate environment promoted health and saved lives.

The third and final story straddles New York City and its seashore. It also highlights the public's captivation with children's health within specific environments. In 1904, a small boy named Joe Marion left his home in the city and traveled to Sea Breeze, a hospital in Coney Island that cared for children with tuberculosis. Joe had a particularly bad case of the disease: his spine was so twisted he could barely walk. In keeping with the treatment regimen of the time, physicians bound Joe to a curved board to help straighten his spine. Despite his condition, Joe was known for his cherubic grin. An appeal for money informed readers that Joe was "crippled by bone tuberculosis, strapped to a board night and day." Yet, readers also learned that Joe "smiles because he is being wonderfully cured at Sea Breeze, by the outdoor salt air treatment, the first American temporary hospital for such cases."[19] "Smiling Joe" became the poster boy for Sea Breeze. Although the hospital circulated a picture of Joe strapped to a frame, the accompanying text highlighted the importance of the seaside location where Joe resided, informing readers that the sea breeze facilitated the child's recovery. Later his doctors reported that time at the seashore had cured Joe of his condition.

Each of these stories focuses on children's seemingly miraculous recoveries and captures the changing, and even contradictory, medical terrain of the time. As the first two stories suggest, rapid scientific and medical discoveries promised new and efficacious treatments during the late nineteenth and early twentieth centuries. In 1881, Pasteur developed a vaccine for anthrax, a disease that had killed flocks of sheep and infected humans. Shortly thereafter, German physician Robert Koch identified the bacilli that caused tuberculosis and cholera.[20] In 1885, Pasteur developed his treatment for rabies, which was technically a vaccine that could be administered after someone was bitten. The same year, Spanish physician Jaime Ferrán distributed the first vaccine for cholera, giving it to thirty thousand people in Spain.[21] A handful of other innovations emerged, such as a diphtheria antitoxin (1894) and diagnostic tests for tuberculosis and syphilis.

Over the first half of the twentieth century, scientists, physicians, and technicians developed new drugs that improved some outcomes; notable among those drugs was insulin, which transformed diabetes from a fatal to a chronic condition.[22] As the tale about baby incubator shows indicates, the public was captivated by technological advances and their potential to save lives. While most patients still preferred to receive medical treatment within their homes, by the early twentieth century hospitals had become an important locus of care.[23] Urban institutions boasted the latest technologies, including x-rays and gleaming sterile surgical environments.[24]

Despite these profound shifts in medicine, Smiling Joe's story indicates that physicians continued to celebrate the beach as a therapeutic landscape. Germ theory and laboratory methods may have given rise to new technologies and ideas regarding the cause of disease, but they provided little insight into the mechanisms of health and well-being.[25] This allowed physicians to continue to use the seashore as a site of care and cure.

Curing and Caring for Patients at the Seashore

As noted above, seaside tourism and marine medication fit within practices of traveling for health. In the mid-nineteenth century, French physician André Brochard advocated for his system of "marine medication." He penned his experiences, publishing *Sea-Air and Sea-Bathing for Children and Invalids: Their Properties, Uses, and Modes of Employment* in 1864. The book was an international success. By 1865, British physician William Strange had translated it from French into English, and by the early 1870s it had made its way across the Atlantic Ocean and into the hands of the men who founded the Children's Seashore House in Atlantic City, New Jersey.[26]

Brochard reported that time at the seashore improved the health of children suffering from a vast range of conditions, including scrofula (tuberculosis of the glands), debility, afflictions of the stomach and bowels, rapid or slow growth, worms, chronic bronchitis, nervous excitability, and "disease of spoiled children."[27] This outcome would have impressed colleagues, given the dearth of targeted treatments or cures for such conditions.

Even more promisingly, other physicians replicated Brochard's results. In 1870, British physician George Oliver published an article in the *British Medical Journal* that outlined eight groups of patients who improved while on England's northeast coast. This included people suffering from active childhood diseases, scrofula, some functional disorders of the nervous system, dyspepsia, tissue degeneration, "hay-asthma," and debility. The seashore, Oliver claimed, also benefited patients who were convalescing.[28]

Reading these lists of illnesses that marine medication supposedly cured can raise skepticism, especially given twenty-first-century understandings of disease causation. Many conditions sound vague, and some no longer exist as diagnostic categories. Moreover, how could so many patients with such different diseases all benefit from simply going to the beach?

Yet marine medication was not fringe, and its practitioners were not hucksters or snake-oil salesmen. Elite physicians on both sides of the Atlantic promoted the practice.[29] Oliver's study appeared in the *British Medical Journal*, one of the most prestigious medical publications in the Western world. Medical conferences dedicated entire sessions to discussing the seashore's healing properties. Highly trained physicians opened and staffed seashore hospitals along Europe's coasts and the northeastern coast of the United States. Urban doctors referred patients to the institutions, and at least one city-based hospital, St. Christopher's in Philadelphia, opened as the winter annex for a seaside institution.[30]

Physicians, patients, and knowledge flowed between urban centers and the seashore, establishing the beach as a site that could cure diseases that thrived in urban areas. Debility is a prime example. Today we no longer have a diagnostic category for debility but generally think of it as, per the *Cambridge Dictionary*, a "physical weakness." Debility had a far more robust definition in the nineteenth and early twentieth centuries.[31] In 1870, Oliver characterized debility as a state when "expenditure of energy has exceeded the supply; exhaustion has occurred, and will continue, until income and expenditure are again fairly balanced."[32] In an article published in the American Medical Association's journal almost thirty years later, American physician John Robison defined debility as a condition marked by "anemia, malaise, loss of flesh and strength, insomnia, nervous irritability, and similar symptoms."[33]

Medical professionals claimed that city life induced a debilitated state. In 1870, Oliver discursively tied the two together when noting patients who had "debility produced by Town life" benefited from time at England's shore. The staff at the Children's Seashore House echoed this sentiment in 1882 when they defined debility as "incident to the hot weather and a crowded city."[34] If urban environments caused debility, then it followed that removing patients from the city was not just beneficial but necessary for healing.

Oliver further knit debility to urban life by linking the condition to overstimulation, which physicians believed cities induced. Turning his attention to other conditions, Oliver underscored that the "tonic properties of sea-air are of great value to those persons whose energies are exhausted by overwork, especially of the brain, or by what is commonly called worry."[35] Sea air restored energy and calmed nerves. He also argued that sea air and sea-bathing increased patients' appetites and strengthened weak patients. According to Oliver, this result was valuable to those with debility, as well as patients who needed to gain weight, such as children and convalescents.[36]

Physicians also promoted the notion that the seashore strengthened the debilitated bodies of adults and children. At least one seashore hospital dedicated a large portion of its beds to patients diagnosed with debility. In the summer of 1887, nearly 200 of the 500 patients who arrived at the Children's Seashore House in Atlantic City suffered from debility.[37] This trend accelerated into the twentieth century. In 1910, 1,596 of the facility's 2,547 patients, or more than 62 percent, had debility; head lice and tuberculosis were the next most common conditions, with 97 patients having the former condition and 97 the latter.[38]

Doctors continued to claim that the seashore cured an incredible range of maladies. In 1887, the Children's Seashore House treated 502 children and 154 mothers.[39] In 1910, after moving to a larger building, it admitted 2,547 children and 364 mothers, while welcoming 278 boys to its summer camp.[40] That year supporters of the Children's Seashore House learned that the beachside hospital treated patients with everything from scrapes, burns, rashes, and broken bones, to paralysis, tuberculosis, and nephritis. At the facility, the number of conditions treated expanded in comparison to the nineteenth-century patient logs. In one year, physicians and nurses admitted patients with the following diagnoses:

> abrasions of the head, hand and knee; abscess; adenitis; adenoids, amputation, anemia, arthritis, ascaris lumbucoides, asthma; appendicitis, athetosis, burn, bronchitis, broncho-pneumonia, cholera infantum, chorea, congenital dislocation of the hip; conjunctivitis; contusions, cretinism, convalescent, debility, dentition, dysentery, dysmenorrhea,

> diphtheria, eczema, endocarditis, enuresis, empyema, epilepsy, enterocolitis, erythema multiforme, felon, fibrosities of plantar fascia; fracture, furunculosis, gastritis, gastro-enteritis, genu valgum, heat prostration, hernia, hypertrophied tonsils, hypospadias, inanition, infection, insomnia, kyphosis, keratitis, laceration, malnutrition, mastoiditis, metrorrhagia, muscular contraction, necrosis, nephritis, nervousness, organic heart disease, osteomyelitis, otitis media, ovaritis, ozena, prolapsus ani, paralysis, pediculosis capitis, pharyngitis, pseudomeningitis, rheumatism, scoliosis, struma, taenia saginata, tertian malaria, traumatic knee, tuberculosis, varicella.[41]

New views of disease causation, brought about by germ theory, did little to quell popular or medical support for marine medication, even into the early twentieth century.

Doctors did acknowledge, however, that marine medication could not cure everyone.[42] They argued that while the seashore benefited children with tuberculosis of the joints or lymph nodes, it could harm patients who suffered from pulmonary tuberculosis.[43] Oliver claimed that the northeastern coast of England at Redcar and Saltburn aggravated the conditions of patients with all stages of tubercular consumption (pulmonary tuberculosis). Physicians attributed this to the region's fluctuating temperatures and sea winds, which could compound problems for patients with lung disease.[44]

American physicians largely agreed, although some believed time at the shore could help adult patients with early-stage pulmonary TB. In 1884, Atlantic City physician Boardman Reed argued that Atlantic City's climate could benefit pulmonary tuberculosis patients before the disease fully developed. He presented the case of an eighteen-year-old patient as proof. The young woman traveled from New York City to Atlantic City in the spring of 1882. After arriving in Atlantic City, she saw a local physician, who determined her to be in the early stages of consumption. The patient's health improved over the subsequent month at the beach. She gained weight and built her strength, and her cough subsided. She left the seaside town, traveled to the mountains, then back to New York City, and finally returned to Atlantic City the following spring. At the seashore her doctor lamented that his patient now had "profuse purulent expectoration, with high fever." Her tuberculosis had worsened. Unlike on her previous visit, on this trip the seashore exacerbated her condition, and the patient's health deteriorated quickly. She died three weeks after her arrival.[45]

In contrast to adults, doctors discovered that tubercular children flourished at the shore. Young patients with nonpulmonary forms of tuberculosis showed remarkable improvements after moving from the city to the beach; their abscesses closed, spines straightened, and joints became mobile. Doctors considered these transformations to be "almost miraculous."[46] In an article included in the 1882 annual report for the Children's Seashore House, the author argued that for boys and girls who had "known scrofulous tendencies . . . sea air is the best possible tonic, and a stay at this institution often decides in their favor the question whether they shall grow up cripples or overcome the disease lurking in them and become strong men and women."[47]

Urban-based practitioners also recognized the rehabilitative benefits of the seashore. On May 14, 1895, DeForest Willard, a preeminent and pioneering orthopedic surgeon in Philadelphia, wrote a letter to William Bennett, the physician in charge of the Children's Seashore House.[48] Having reviewed the facility's results, Willard concluded, "Your circular of the Sea-Shore House is at hand, offering its beneficial and much appreciated aid in the work of restoring crippled children to health. I know of no Association which has done more good work, or that has obtained better results than this one. May we ask again for the favor of sending about a dozen children to the Home from the University Wards and Dispensary? If so, will you kindly send blanks?"[49] Perhaps Willard needed space in his unit, but his letter reveals his willingness to use the seashore as a place to rehabilitate children with orthopedic conditions, caused by diseases like tuberculosis and rickets. It also indicates that elite physicians embraced the seashore's healing potential. Often children whose health conditions remained resistant to treatment in cities recovered once they moved to the beach. Their reformed bodies offered visual proof of the seashore's salubrious results.

Bodies of Evidence

In 1911, two boys arrived at the Children's Seashore House from a Philadelphia-based hospital. Their city physician was frustrated with their lack of improvement. He sent a note to his colleagues at the seashore facility telling them that the boys should "be forced to eat." That intervention never came to pass. The staff at the seaside hospital reported that the boys' "awakened seashore appetite demanded double helpings at their first breakfast and soon they were brown, round and hungry as sturdy whistling country boys."[50]

These boys were not anomalies; many children gained weight and a tan after a stay at the seashore. Children who left cities pale and weak returned to their urban homes bronzed and strong. Their bodily changes reinforced health claims that the seashore restored what cities depleted. Numerical data supported corporeal evidence. Doctors pointed to children's weight gain as measurable proof of marine medication's efficacy.[51] In 1884, Boardman Reed wrote that sea air's benefits included "a general tonic influence with increased appetite."[52] Doctors at seashore hospitals reported that pediatric patients gained significant amounts of weight, and their physicians provided charts that documented children's ages, diagnoses, lengths of stay, and weight at admission and discharge.[53] They reminded the public that since many of the children were admitted from urban hospitals, patients' improvements could not be explained by improved sanitary conditions or better nutrition. The beach environment, rather than hospital-based care or nutrition, made the difference.

Patients' improvements bolstered physicians' claims that the beach could cure. The results also inspired doctors to consider whether a winter spent at the beach could also benefit patients. In the United States, physicians had initially limited their recommendation of travel to the northeastern seashore to the summer months. After decades of practice, however, they expanded their prescription to include wintertime stays. In their view, a prolonged residence during the winter was especially beneficial for children with chronic orthopedic conditions.

The Children's Seashore House dabbled in wintertime care as early as 1883, but few patients applied for admission at first.[54] Interest grew in the twentieth century. In 1917, William Bennett, the long-standing physician in charge of the Children's Seashore House, celebrated the seashore's year-round rehabilitative properties. He described how medical providers delighted in watching "children growing ruddy and strong as they lie on their beds on the porches, or swiftly hobble on their crutches over the beach" during the winter months. His staff was preoccupied by the fact that so much of their institution lay empty for the majority of the year. They claimed they could fill 120 beds during the winter, arguing that the hospital could "be occupied by other children at present in their little, unsanitary homes or the City Hospital wards, who, if we had the means, might also be growing ruddy and strong in our sunshine and sea air."[55] Bennett planted the image of children frolicking on the beach to advocate for expanding the hospital's work. He positioned the seaside as a place where children could heal and relax in the open air and play on the beach, instead of remaining immobilized in "unsanitary" homes, regardless of the season.

Seashore hospitals also contrasted urban pediatric institutions in the types of care they could provide. Practitioners at seashore hospitals centered treatment on movement in, and exposure to, the natural surroundings rather than primarily relying on surgery. Seaside institutions, including Sea Breeze, founded in 1904 on Coney Island, and Crawford Allen Hospital, a beachfront hospital founded outside of Providence, Rhode Island, in 1906, are illustrative of this trend. Both hospitals admitted children with orthopedic conditions, including tuberculosis, polio, and osteomyelitis, a bone infection.[56] Albert Miller, a physician at Crawford Allen, argued that while restrictive orthopedic interventions, such as braces, splints, casts, and immobilization, reduced "deformities of those patients who have survived, [they have] had little effect in lessening the suffering and fatality of the disease."[57] Physicians in urban hospitals treated tuberculosis of the bones and joints with operations. Following surgery, physicians would immobilize a patient's affected limb or joint with instruments like braces, splints, and plaster casts.[58]

Patients' experiences at seashore hospitals starkly contrasted their time in city institutions. Children at Crawford Allen spent their days and nights in the open air and enjoyed "freedom from restraint, both mental and physical."[59] Patients at the shore still might need casts or braces, but rather than performing surgery or restraining patients, seaside medical professionals encouraged patients' active lifestyles. Even children in braces and plaster jackets participated in sea bathing. Children who required hip braces were outfitted with removable devices held together with straps, while patients in plaster jackets were allowed to wade in the shallow water.[60] Children at Crawford Allen wrestled and played baseball and other games, although physicians and nurses tried to keep affected joints "quiet."[61]

Physicians offered statistical evidence of the seashore's tonic influence. Over a single summer at Crawford Allen, Miller reported that twelve patients arrived either bedridden or wheelchair bound, thirteen required crutches, and just seven walked unaided. By the end of the summer, only two children returned to urban hospital wards (presumably bedridden), two were in beds or wheelchairs, eighteen on crutches, and twelve walked without assistance. He reported that patients' weight and joint mobility increased. All the children's open wounds improved and some healed entirely. Despite the limited scope of his trial, Miller argued that these outcomes supported marine medication and "freedom from unnecessary restraint" as effective treatments.[62] His patients' bodies provided visible and quantifiable measures of marine medication's superlative benefits in contrast to the outcomes seen in urban institutions.

Sea Breeze in Coney Island also relied on marine medication to care for its patients.[63] However, its physicians did utilize techniques that restricted patients' movement more than did their counterparts at Crawford Allen. For example, physicians at Sea Breeze prescribed bed rest for acute cases and immobilized patients or placed them in traction, practices that differed from those of their northern neighbors. In addition, patients at Sea Breeze always remained in their orthopedic devices, which meant that patients with hip disease were typically unable to go swimming.[64] The physician in charge allowed one patient with hip tuberculosis to enter the sea to ameliorate a particularly "offensive discharge from the sinuses." That child wore a specially designed removable cast, which he took off to bathe. The patient's results were so encouraging that physician B. H. Whitbeck decided to use similar casts for more patients the following summer, but he intended to modify them with rubber so that patients could swim in them.[65]

Physicians agreed that the marine environment improved pediatric patients' mobility. In 1911, Roland Hammond, a prominent orthopedic surgeon affiliated with Crawford Allen, noted that many colleagues considered the seashore climate to be superior to that of urban and even rural hospitals. Orthopedic surgeons argued that the composition of the sea air, the invigorating effects of seawater, and outdoor life promoted patients' improvement. Hammond commented that through the combination of environmental conditions, as well as "the best of food, and the comradeship of other happy children, the opsonic index is raised and nature is provided with her best weapons for fighting these diseases."[66] When Hammond invoked the opsonic index—the degree to which bacteria are susceptible to being consumed or eliminated by other cells—he tied marine medication's work to bacteriological models of disease and to germ theory. In doing so he grounded marine medication's results in the scientific metrics that localized health within the body, rather than outside of it.

Hammond was not alone; other marine medication advocates in the early twentieth century were also caught up in the current of laboratory-produced medical knowledge. These physicians *knew* that marine medication worked and had published data and quantitative evidence of patients' results. But physicians wanted to know why. Were there specific elements that made the beach beneficial? If so, what were they? Asking these questions led physicians to bring the seashore into the lab and under the lens of scientific scrutiny.

Making Marine Medication Scientific

Marine medication included a combination of sea air, seawater, and sun exposure. Indeed, if we could visit the Children's Seashore House in the 1870s and then time-travel sixty years into the future, patients' medical care would look much the same. You would see patients whiling away their days on the beach. They would sit on porches and in the sand, take brief sea baths, and play under the sun.

If instead you flipped through medical journals, the difference would be more pronounced. Physicians in the early twentieth century still promoted the myriad benefits of marine medication and advocated for sea air, seawater, and sunbathing. However, they increasingly reduced and rationalized environmental therapeutics. By the twentieth century, marine medication practitioners were conducting comparative studies of children's metabolism in different environments, measuring their oxidation levels, recording IQs, and creating and consulting radiographic images for visual and numerical evidence of healing. This approach aligned marine medication with professional trends, and it gave scientific credibility to "balneotherapy" (swimming), "heliotherapy," (sunbathing), and sea-air baths.[67]

SEAWATER

Physicians regulated balneotherapy from the beginning of marine medication, while nurses controlled and monitored patients' bathing practices. Swimming at the Children's Seashore House exemplified the precision of a physician's dosing. In 1875, the resident physician at the facility designated 11:00 a.m. as the bathing hour. He permitted children to sea-bathe between three and seven days a week depending on their age, health, and general constitution. Nurses designated a spot in the ocean, and ambulatory children waded into the waves. Once in the water, the children bobbed up and down, dunking themselves beneath the ocean's surface.

We also know that medical professionals believed that children, particularly those who were weak and ill, could be harmed by unregulated bathing. Across time, physicians cautioned that staying in the water too long was dangerous.[68] Doctors warned bathers about the progressive reactions they would experience and the consequences of bathing with abandon. Marine medication advocate André Brochard defined the first reaction as the "phenomena of immersion."[69] His description evokes a visceral memory for anyone who has taken a polar plunge or bathed in the cold waters of the Atlantic.[70] Brochard characterized the various phenomena of immersion as "a sensation of cold, often sharp, sometimes even painful; immediately followed by a general spasm. The skin is chilled, it becomes pale, puckered, like the skin of fowls, sometimes blue. . . . The breathing is catching; if the bather tries to speak, his words are ejaculated one by one; a trembling seizes the jaws and limbs, and the pulse becomes small and thready."[71] Pleasure was the reward for the initial shock. Brochard called this second phase the "phenomena of reaction." During this period bathers experienced a sense of expansion or invigoration, which physicians characterized by a return of warmth, as well as regular breathing, a decrease in heart rate, a full pulse, and rosy skin.[72] Depending on the bather's age, health, and constitution, this phase of reaction could last several minutes.

Doctors warned their patients and one another that it was imperative for bathers to remove themselves from the ocean before the second phase subsided. Staying in the ocean too long resulted in the return of the symptoms of the "phenomena of immersion," but to a potentially harmful extent. When this occurred, patients' systems could become depressed, causing "coma, syncope, throbbing headache, apoplexy in the aged, congestion of the internal organs, subnormal temperature, or death."[73] To avoid these ill effects, physicians at the Children's Sea House limited their patients' ocean baths to a maximum of four minutes, warning that longer exposure diminished their health.[74]

When patients sea-bathed correctly, they enjoyed a variety of health benefits. Doctors hypothesized that the shock of the initial immersion forced internal organs to release warm blood, which then traveled to the surface of the body, thereby increasing circulation. They concluded that this sequence improved the quality and quantity of the patient's blood; helped respiration become deeper, longer, and more regular; increased appetite; made skin become firmer, warmer, and rosy; and helped the patient sleep more soundly.[75]

The benefits could be great, but the dangers were real. Not all patients were strong enough to withstand the waves and the tides. Seashore hospitals employed "bathers" to assist these patients. Bathers, usually men, would place young and weak children on a chair, in a stretcher, or in a basket and carry them into the ocean to bathe. Given the medical argument about the need to strictly control exposure to ocean water, the bather's job was likely understood to be potentially hazardous.

In photographs of the bathers and their charges, it is unclear why the young men chose, or were chosen, to be bathers. One possible explanation is that the public did not adhere to the same beliefs as the medical profession about the potentially harmful effects of sea-bathing. We know that physicians lamented this reality.[76] Another possibility is that medical professionals saw these men as either expendable or able to withstand the effects of sea-bathing, perhaps due to their ethnicity, race, or general health. Given the dedication of the

Children's Sea House to serving patients and families from all races, which archival records and photographs support, the latter seems a less compelling conclusion.

Bathers continued to bring patients into the waves in the twentieth century, and the practices of sea-bathing remained strikingly consistent for more than seventy years. Sir Henry Gauvain, a British physician, also advocated for sea-bathing as a treatment for patients with surgical tuberculosis, although he used more scientific language to explain the effects.[77] In 1933, Gauvain described patients' reactions to entering the ocean: "On immersion the patient experiences a cold shock . . . there is superficial vaso-constriction, and heat is rapidly abstracted from the body. The child generally involuntarily gasps for breath."[78] Gauvain claimed that the ensuing "rapid and deep respiration" was beneficial because it "increased oxygenation of the tissues with a correspondingly greater elimination of CO_2." He concluded that short baths were necessary in the beginning of a patient's treatment but that "later a longer period is required in the water—to the evident enjoyment of the child."[79]

Physicians' justification for sea-bathing became more scientific sounding, but their concerns with dosing remained. In 1922, physicians at the Hayling Island branch of Lord Mayor Treloar Hospital in England limited patients' bathing to intervals of thirty seconds to seven minutes during the summer months.[80] Doctors would also have patients acclimate to sea baths. Patients would paddle into seawater for an increasing amount of time, endure seawater sprays, and finally submerge themselves beneath the surf. As in previous decades, children immersed themselves under nurses' watchful gaze, or an attendant carried patients into the water.

By the twentieth century, physicians at Hayling Island were advocating for balneotherapy, claiming it increased muscle tone and encouraged patients to breathe deeper, which improved circulation. By extending or limiting patients' time in the ocean, physicians also used sea-bathing to alter and control a patient's metabolism.[81] Physicians Leonard Hill, J. Argyll Campbell, and Gauvain wrote that, by altering the time children spent bathing, physicians had "a ready and controllable means of stimulating metabolism to a desired degree."[82] By dosing ocean bathing, physicians titrated patients' reactions to yield measurable results.

SEA AIR

Individuals at the shore spent the majority of their time outside in the sea air and sea breeze, whether they were patients at a seashore hospital or private citizens at the beach. Sea air exposure fit with prevailing medical advice in the late nineteenth and early twentieth centuries. Physicians and public health officials stressed that outdoor life and fresh air benefited all patients, but they placed special emphasis on the positive outcomes for the urban poor and tuberculosis sufferers.[83] They argued that the marine climate induced change because it contrasted the "devitalized air of large cities" from which patients came.[84]

Unlike the city's foul, stagnant, and putrid air, sea breezes were fresh, pure, and laden with ozone and saline particles. Since the discovery of ozone, a reactive and unstable gas that consists of three oxygen atoms (O_3) instead of the usual two (O_2), in the mid-nineteenth century, scientists and physicians had believed that it purified the air. Scientific studies found little or no presence of ozone in cities, particularly during epidemics. In contrast, they detected an abundance of it in regions like the seashore and mountains. These studies led physicians to conclude that ozone made air fresh and healthy.[85]

Physicians also argued that sea air was healthy because it lacked disease-causing particles. In 1884, Boardman Reed argued that the near constant motion of sea-air meant that it was free from both "noxious effluvia" and bacteria.[86] Reed's statement offers insight into a moment of transition during which physicians blended miasmatic and bacteriological theories to support environmental therapeutic systems.[87] Under the new rubric, the sea breeze benefited patients by removing disease-causing agents and by surrounding patients with health-enhancing ozone.

Physicians expected multiple tonic effects from sea air exposure. In the same article, Reed argued that ozone unquestionably enhances "the vigor and activity of all the vital processes."[88] According to Reed, as people traveled from the city to the shore, they experienced an increase in air density, causing them to inhale more air, which contained more ozone. This change, he argued, resulted in greater oxidation of the blood and improved bodily functions.[89] Physicians also determined that sea air was beneficial because it was impregnated with alkaline saline particles.

Scientists grounded sea air's curative capabilities in investigations of its chemical composition, density, and movement.[90] Physicians' identification of ozone as a specific health-giving element legitimated marine medication within the reductionist rubric of scientific medicine in the late nineteenth and early twentieth centuries. That view also disintegrated sea air, rendering it less about the sea breeze and more about the invisible particles that entered one's lungs and altered bodily systems and responses.

SUNLIGHT

Sunlight in specific doses was the final addition to marine medication in the United States. In the twentieth century, medical practitioners conceived of sunbathing as a medical intervention, not just a popular practice. Swiss physician Auguste Rollier devised a natural sunbathing system at his alpine sanitarium. Nurses dispensed doses of sunshine by gradually exposing patients' bodies to the light. On the first day, they would wheel patients onto sunporches and then pull back the sheets to expose patients' feet. After five minutes, nurses replaced the covers. From that day on, nurses performed a ritual of daily sunbathing.[91] On day two, a patient's calves joined the feet for the dose of sun. Feet felt the sun's rays for ten-minute bursts, while the calves were permitted only five minutes of sunbathing. Day by day nurses revealed more body parts for longer periods. This practice continued until the patient was tan and acclimated to the sun.

Using sunlight to treat patients was not a new idea in the early twentieth century. However, physicians differentiated their system from previous practices by dosing sunlight and tying heliotherapy to bacteriology. Doctors referenced studies of sunlight's bactericidal properties to explain why it worked. Scientists had determined that UV rays killed bacteria and molds.[92] Doctors reasoned that, if UV rays killed bacteria, it followed that sunlight could heal infected wounds and be used to treat patients with bacterial diseases such as tuberculosis. Not only did the sun turn patients into sturdy, tanned children, but it also became a weapon in medicine's bactericidal arsenal.[93]

Physicians quantified sunbathing's physiological impact as well. In 1912, the Crawford Allen Hospital adopted "the all-over sun bath in all cases of bone disease."[94] The hospital administrators paid for a sun deck that they outfitted

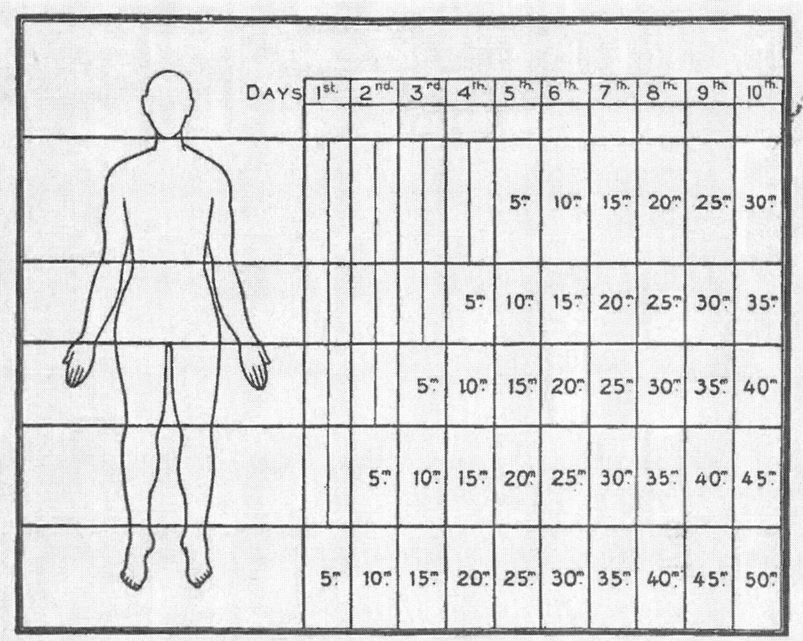

FIGURE 4. Chart that shows the schedule for progressive natural sunbathing or "heliotherapy." Auguste Rollier, *Heliotherapy* (London: Henry Frowde and Hodder & Stoughton, 1923), 23.

with windscreens and small sunshades to protect the children's heads from becoming too hot. As in Switzerland, attendants wheeled patients outside so they could sunbathe. Hammond quantified the results. He compared patients' weight gain and hemoglobin levels from 1911 and 1912. He reported that children who received heliotherapy and balneotherapy rather than just bathing in the sea experienced a greater increase in average weight (4.2 pounds versus 3 pounds) and hemoglobin levels (17 percent versus 0.8 percent increase). Hammond claimed that patients were healthier in the spring of 1913 than in any previous year, despite spending winters in the city.[95] Hammond had quantitative evidence that heliotherapy bolstered children's health and resistance to urban conditions.

Other doctors documented the sun's influence on intelligence. Working with a colleague, Gauvain studied the mental capacities of pediatric patients in hospitals in Alton and Hayling Island in England. The physicians observed that children who received heliotherapy had 10 percent higher mental intelligence than those who did not. Physicians concluded that heliotherapy increased patients' "potentialities and prospects."[96] Although Gauvain's assertion seemed to align with eugenicists' goals, they have more in common with "euthenics," a program that promoted race betterment through environmental intervention, rather than programs of selective breeding.[97] Moreover, Albert Miller of the Crawford Allen acknowledged that treatment of "crippled" patients may seem to work against eugenic principles, but he argued that marine medication alleviated these children's suffering. He implored his colleagues to "unite in believing that any time spent in freeing their distorted little bodies from suffering is time well spent."[98]

Over decades of practicing marine medication, physicians increasingly distilled, dosed, and applied sunlight, sea air, and seawater to care for patients. Doing so shifted beliefs about why the seashore was salubrious. Their scientific approaches operated like blinders: physicians and patients could no longer look at the expansive beachscape and see bodies cured and reformed by a healthy environment. Rather, the seashore was a syringe that injected a dose of medicine, which bodies absorbed in specific pathways to produce quantifiable results.

IN 1912, the physician in charge of the Children's Seashore House could still wax poetic about the transformative power of the seaside. William Bennett celebrated that his patients' "hearty appetites, rosy cheeks and rounded limbs attest to all the value of this method of Nature's cure, while physicians, accustomed to the slow progress which takes places in these chronic ailments, look often with surprise upon the changes wrought in their little patients by their residence by the sea."[99] Bennett proffered patients' physical changes as proof of the seashore's therapeutic value.

Yet his words also hint at the beginnings of a rift between urban and seashore practitioners. Bennett had practiced marine medication for four decades. He knew it worked because he saw it every day. Yet his Philadelphia-based colleagues expressed "surprise" at their patients' recoveries. In 1912, city practitioners were still willing to prescribe marine medication, but some did not anticipate it would be so beneficial. Early twentieth-century practitioners, particularly those who grew up with and trained in bacteriology, embraced a different view of health, bodies, and the environment. Rather than promoting the curative effect of place, they celebrated the elements it harbored.

The seashore had become a sum of its parts.[100] Ozone-rich air oxidized the blood, while the seawater's minerals cleansed young patients' sores, and the sun's UV rays killed bacteria that lived in and on those wounds. The more physicians sought to rationalize the marine environment, the harder it became to conceptualize the seashore as holistically salubrious.

Physicians reduced the once therapeutic landscape to invisible tonic elements. Although the practices of marine medication looked largely the same in the 1920s and 1930s as they had in the 1860s and 1870s, the scientific knowledge that supported sending children to the beach limited medical understanding about why the beach was beneficial. By the 1920s, the seashore had transitioned from a therapeutic landscape to a mechanism to expose patients to discrete and quantifiable healthy elements.

THREE THE SHIFTING SANDS OF HEALTH TOURISM

IN THE MID-NINETEENTH CENTURY, Dr. Jonathan Pitney stood on the sands of Absecon Island and scanned the shore. The barrier island sat just off the coast of New Jersey, and at the time it was little more than windswept sand, sea grass, and prickly bushes clinging to the dunes. A handful of homes studded the otherwise sparse landscape. Most visitors who came to the island saw nothing more than "an arid waste of sand."[1] Pitney, however, envisioned a grand health resort.

Just fifty years later Atlantic City was a bustling seaside town.[2] Far from a barren landscape, the beach was crowded with hotels, piers, restaurants, and attractions that filled the skyline. A five-mile boardwalk acted as a permeable boundary that separated the built from the natural environment.[3] Hundreds of thousands of visitors came during the summer to the so-called City by the Sea to frequent movie houses, sideshows, and carnival rides that lined the western side of the boardwalk.[4] While in Atlantic City, tourists could see Jim Key the educated horse or seek the vertiginous merry-go-rounds, mazes, and Ferris wheels.[5] Those in the mood for something particularly dramatic could watch a reenactment of the Johnstown flood, a tragic event that killed over twenty-two hundred people in 1889 when a dam burst and water roared down a valley to engulf the western Pennsylvania city.

Tourists also came for the beach. Swimmers clutched the safety ropes that led them into the sea, and the ocean became bloated with bathers. Men, women, children, and the occasional donkey roamed and lounged on the sands. Tourists whiled away the hours, playing in the surf and enjoying the company of others.

The seashore's popularity fit within larger trends at the time. An increasing

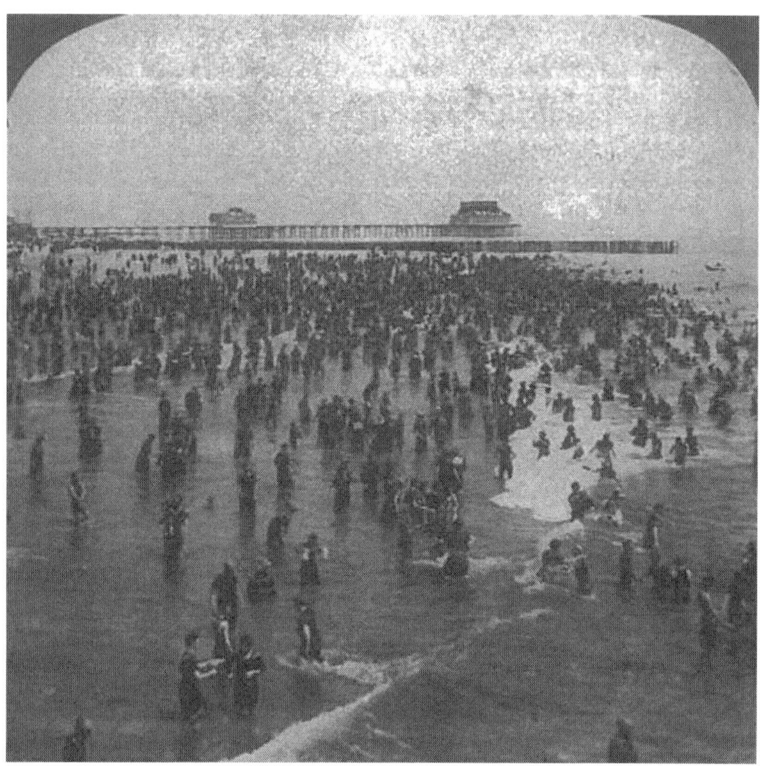

FIGURE 5. Photograph of a beach full of bathers at Atlantic City. Geo. W. Griffith, Publisher, Philadelphia, Pennsylvania. Author's collection.

number of Americans, particularly from the upper and middle classes, began to travel in the nineteenth century. At this time Americans were renegotiating their feelings toward leisure and how travel fit within cultural ethics of work.[6] Traveling for health offered a rationalization for vacations. Restoring health meant being able to labor with greater strength and in better mental spirit. The seashore's therapeutic association made it a morally sound destination, and its popularity accelerated in the twentieth century.

This chapter illuminates the premise that health was a central reason that Americans experienced travel and knew the seashore. By the late nineteenth century, more Americans could spend time at the beach, with railroads transporting greater numbers of urban residents, including those from working-class families. By 1873, approximately half a million tourists were going to Atlantic City every summer.[7] While the beauty of the landscape might have inspired some to travel to the ocean, most seaside tourists went because they understood that they could benefit from and enjoy their time in the healthy environment.

Of course most people did not read medical journal articles about marine medication but instead learned of the seashore's therapeutic value by word of mouth, doctors' prescriptions, or promotional tracts. Newspapers celebrated the seaside resorts' therapeutic success in curing diseases and remedying chronic conditions. Americans learned that sea breezes, saltwater, and sunlight gave the landscape its therapeutic value. With few exceptions, historians have not analyzed health as a primary motivator in the rise of vacations and tourism. Some reference it briefly, others set it aside, and a few dismiss therapeutic claims as outlandish, absurd, or extravagant.[8] But in the nineteenth century, visitors sought and consumed health as a central part of seaside tourism.[9]

This pattern of health-seeking travel continued into the early twentieth century as tourists embraced claims about the relative salubrity of the seashore. However, as we will see, when travelers consumed health care practices and devices, they shifted their travel associations from health to leisure. Visitors toured hospitals, took over bathhouses, and turned wheelchairs into leisure rides and political statements. Marine medication was not only healthy but also entertaining and enjoyable. When visitors used health care practices as pleasurable pursuits, it became harder to associate time at the beach with therapeutic treatments. As we will see, tourists melded leisure and health until they became nearly indistinguishable.

Promoting Healthy Leisure, Popularizing the Shore

Pitney recognized Atlantic City's potential to become a popular health resort, but he needed assistance to transform the beach into a city by the sea. He enlisted Richard Osborne, an engineer in Philadelphia, to develop a plan. Together they convinced prominent businessmen of the island's economic promise. In 1852, Pitney procured a charter for a railroad, sold ten thousand shares of stock in a single day, and began to lay the rails that would connect the shore to nearby Philadelphia.[10]

Osborne promoted Atlantic City as the "lungs of Philadelphia."[11] This was not only a catchy slogan. As noted previously, Frederick Law Olmsted made similar claims about Central Park as the functioning lungs of New York City, meaning it was a space that produced fresh air that (re)invigorated urban residents. Osborne's claims about Atlantic City tapped into prevailing beliefs about cities' stagnant, pestilential air.[12] If fresh air was medicine, the seashore—like a park—could breathe health back into urban residents.

Osborne and Pitney's vision became a reality. In 1854, within two years of the laying of the initial rail, the first train delivered passengers to what would become Atlantic City. The tourists had traveled sixty miles from Philadelphia and represented a who's who of visitors, including reporters and elite members of Philadelphia society. When they arrived, the future seaside resort remained rudimentary, with few amenities along the beach. But a year later, on May 1, 1855, the town's development received a boost when New Jersey's governor approved the charter to create Atlantic City.[13]

At this time some travelers sought "sacred places" that inspired a sense of awe and connection with the vast beauty and grandeur of the American landscape.[14] Awe and health were twin forces. Some of the most prominent figures in US history promoted this association when they advocated for the conservation of American landscapes. In 1865, writing about what would become Yosemite National Park, Olmsted proclaimed that "it is a scientific fact that the occasional contemplation of natural scenes of an impressive character, particularly if this contemplation occurs in connection with relief from ordinary cares, change of air and change of habits, is favorable to the health and vigor of men . . . beyond any other conditions that can be offered them."[15] Over fifty years later, Sierra Club founder John Muir promoted the idea that "everybody needs beauty as well as bread, places to play in and pray in, where Nature may heal and cheer and give strength to body and soul alike."[16] These are the musings of elite men who had the means to promote grand environmental changes that would impact scores of Americans. Crucially, both Olmsted and Muir knit together experiencing and contemplating nature's vastness with increased health, strength, and vigor.

Seaside visitors likely experienced awe at their first sight of the ocean, but that was not the experience that boosters promoted. Rather, the seashore was a space for health, repose, and rejuvenation. It was also meant for masses of urban residents.

Images highlighted the crowded nature of the beach. In August 1873, the popular magazine *Harper's Weekly* published a pencil drawing captioned "The Beach at Atlantic City." It is a busy scene. Mothers in long, high-necked dresses shade themselves with parasols as they watch their children. One mother looks to where her young son points in the waves. Behind her a woman tends to a large child who rests in a perambulator. A blanket covers the child's legs, and the mother adjusts it as an older girl reaches for the child's shoulder. To the left, two young girls sit in the sand, a bucket nestled beside them. One child clutches her doll in her right arm while holding a parasol in the other. A toddler sits beyond them, legs splayed, looking down at the sand. A woman glances over her shoulder at the baby, while a gentleman lounges on the beach, hat removed, holding a cigarette as the smoke wafts in the breeze. Nearby a mustachioed man grasps his cane as he converses with two women. Farther in the distance a family plays croquet, while another woman wades into the ocean with her child. Dogs bound about the beach, one playfully pouncing in the foreground.

Viewers likely recognized suggestions of health, in addition to leisure and play. Shadows cast upon the ladies' faces by their parasols indicate that the sun was abundant. The sea breeze blew, making flags fly at attention and the bows on dresses and hats flutter in the wind. Yet the air flow remained gentle enough that umbrellas did not invert, and babies could happily play without being blasted by sand. Bathhouses and bathers highlight swimming as one of many possible activities. Most of the tourists walk, stand, lounge, or play. The sketch suggests that Atlantic City is a place appropriate for a range of ages and physical abilities.[17]

Harper's Weekly reached hundreds of thousands of readers.[18] Potential tourists learned about the health benefits of the seashore from popular periodicals like it, as well as newspaper reports. When trains whisked Americans from the city and suburbs to the beach, the railroad companies provided riders with promotional literature that highlighted the health benefits, as well as attractions, travelers would find at their destination.[19]

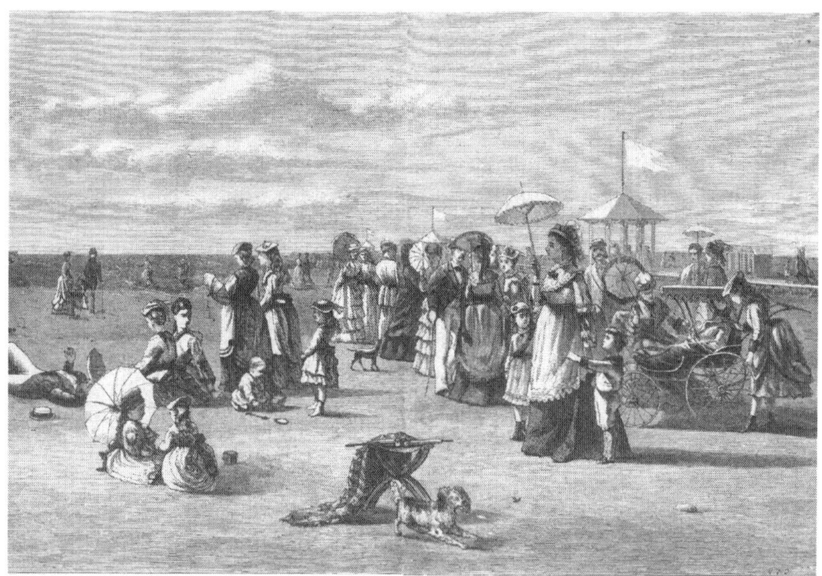

FIGURE 6. A nineteenth-century sketch of tourists engaging in seaside pleasures. Children play while adults tend to their needs, lounge in the sun, and play croquet. "The Beach at Atlantic City," *Harper's Weekly*, August 30, 1873, 764. Accessed via HathiTrust.

The authors of these texts did not make up medical facts.[20] Rather, as we have seen, they tapped into the advanced medical knowledge of the time. As an increasingly large chorus sang the praises of the salubrious sea, the public established new beliefs about the shore. Not long after *Harper's Weekly* published the image of Atlantic City, Philadelphia publisher J. B. Lippincott and Company distributed *Pen and Picture sketches of the City by the Sea*. The 1874 brochure touted the town's health benefits. Readers learned that before the railroad opened, only a handful of people knew Atlantic City's "wonderfully curative powers,—the dry, bracing atmosphere, the cool, delightful breezes that floated over its surface, and the unsurpassed bathing facilities it presented."[21] They learned that "a few enterprising individuals, imbued with a firm faith in its immense value as a seaside resort," established the railroad to facilitate Philadelphians' ability to access the shore town.[22]

Physicians testified to Atlantic City's healthful nature in boosters' promotional materials. Philadelphia physician William V. Keating defined Atlantic City as "one of the most lovely, salubrious climates I have ever visited." He compared Atlantic City's climate to that of Nice, France, and claimed the former "affords relief and cure to all cases of rheumatic fever and arthritis, even in the most acute stages." Placing ocean bathing alongside other water cures, he verified that "many instances in which invalids, after having recourse, without benefit, to the various mineral waters and baths in the country, have there been entirely cured by a summer sojourn" to Atlantic City.[23]

In 1882, physician J. T. King of Baltimore expanded Atlantic City's identity by claiming its value as a summer health resort and a "Winter Sanitarium." In a fifty-page brochure King detailed the benefits of Atlantic City's land and sea breezes, the town's geology, the ocean's color and temperature, the area's climate, its sea air, and its air temperature. King highlighted Atlantic City's "Special Therapeutic Features," which he believed would be "of interest to invalids and physicians."[24] King also solicited feedback from fellow physicians and scientists to support his claims about the health benefits of Atlantic City. Joseph Leidy, famed paleontologist, physician, and professor of anatomy at the University of Pennsylvania, offered his appraisal: "I am pleased to give my testimony as to the health-ness of Atlantic City as a place of resort. I know of no place better adapted to invalids in general." Dr. William Darrach from Germantown, Pennsylvania, concurred: "I cannot recall a case that has not received benefit from a sojourn there. It was of great service in restoring tone to the digestive organs of a case of phthisis during the months of January and February. In the cases of summer complaints in young children marked beneficial results have followed. Convalescents from typhoid fever and bronchial troubles, especially during the spring months, have been completely restored to heath there."[25]

King's pamphlet furthered the association between the seashore and health by introducing readers to the Children's Seashore House, noting that "few of the children who have been admitted to the institution have failed to show, almost immediately, this increase of appetite, and it is, indeed, no exaggeration to say that the effect of the sea-air, in this respect, has been more uniform, and more powerful than that of any therapeutic agent." In addition to improving patients' appetites, King noted, the beach environment allowed patients to experience better sleep, which further facilitated healing. This effect was not limited to patients in hospitals. King argued that even healthy children benefited from the seashore's soporific effects, noting that many children experienced "unusual drowsiness in the daytime, and the afternoon nap becomes an almost irresistible luxury."[26]

These promotional tracts moved medical knowledge out of professional journals and into public discourse. Before the railroads made passage more affordable and faster, middle- and working-class families seldom had the means or time for a sojourn to the sea, but new train routes facilitated families' access to seaside health resorts.[27] Not only was travel to the coast becoming relatively easy, but it could also be done in the name of health. When tourists arrived at the seashore, they found they could witness, and experience health care practices, from taking tours of hospitals, to swimming in the ocean and stopping at bathhouses, and even riding in wheelchairs.

Touring Health

Seashore hospitals were not only physical representations of Americans' beliefs about the health benefits of beach vacations; they were also tourist attractions. The Children's Seashore House was one of Atlantic City's most popular draws. Brochures like King's encouraged people to visit, as did newspapers. In 1875, over two thousand people went to the hospital to tour the institution and its grounds. Visitors continued to trek to the hospital through the first decades of the twentieth century. As late as 1920, tourists came from Rhode Island, Massachusetts, Illinois, Missouri, Ohio, Virginia, Michigan, Colorado, West Virginia, South Carolina, Kentucky, Minnesota, Iowa, North Carolina, Tennessee, and Washington, DC, and even from as far away as Canada, England, and India.[28]

This practice mirrored a popular interest in viewing health care institutions, practices, and patients. Americans frequently toured hospitals and health exhibits in the nineteenth and early twentieth centuries. Some tourists even visited mental health institutions, which shared seashore hospitals' commitment to offering a peaceful, beautiful outdoor environment to promote health and well-being.[29] Other Americans entered their children into Better

Babies contests that evaluated and celebrated healthy youngsters, or Fitter Family contests that gave prizes to large, genetically robust families.[30] As previously detailed, Atlantic City offered several such spectacles, including a baby incubator exhibit where tourists could watch nurses and doctors care for premature infants.[31]

Medical institutions invited the attention. Ideally, tourists would support their work through testimonials and become patrons. Financial support was critical for the success of charity hospitals like the Children's Seashore House and Sea Breeze. Both institutions depended on donations for their operation. Tours served an additional function: they reinforced the idea of the beach as a therapeutic environment. Visitors witnessed children in various states of health and rehabilitation. When tourists lined the fence along Sea Breeze in Coney Island, they could watch weak or disabled children resting in the sea air, while able-bodied children frolicked in the sand. Seeing was believing, and tourists saw that popular activities like sea bathing and sunbathing were therapeutic.[32]

An article published by the *Philadelphia Inquirer* on July 3, 1880, highlighted this association. The author recommended a visit to the Children's Seashore House and asserted that there was "no better way of celebrating the Fourth . . . than a trip to the city by the sea, with a generous contribution to be left in passing at this admirable institution." Visitors would be "enlightened as to its character . . . by the very pretty spectacle, which, during most hours of the day, the small inmates present as they disport themselves on the sand or in the sea. For the latter healthful pastime the children are divided into three classes. The first two bathing thrice a week, the third going in daily for a tumble in the surf. The bathing is always done under the vigilant supervision of faithful nurses."[33] Nurses' presence underscored that sea air, seawater, and sunbathing were therapeutic regimens that required medical supervision.[34] Seeing it firsthand confirmed that time at the beach was healthy.

Buildings also communicated that the beach could cure. Architects designed beachfront hospitals to maximize exposure to the seashore's medicinal environment. The first building of the Children's Seashore House, finished in the 1870s, had a "wide and roomy piazza [that] extends around the ground floor of the entire building, the roof of which serves as a balcony for the second

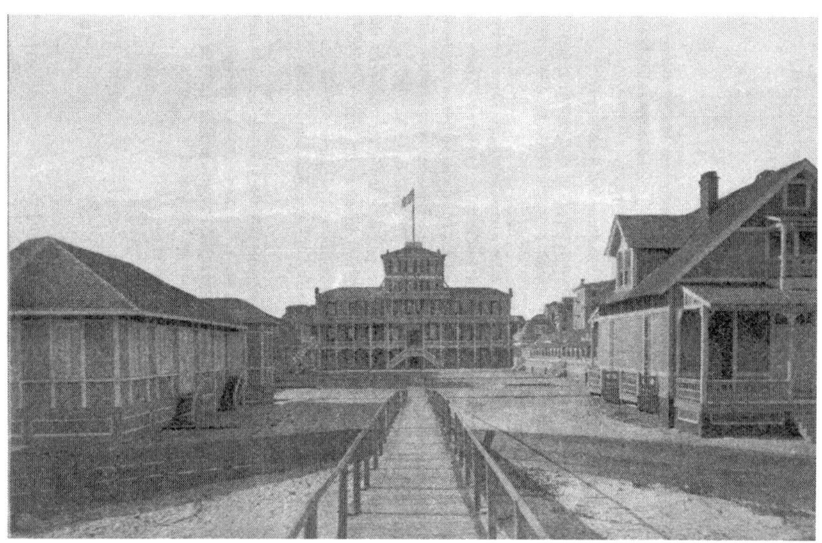

FIGURE 7. Photograph of the Children's Seashore House's first permanent hospital building, 1870s. The main building is a large wooden structure flanked by mothers' cottages. *Children's Seashore House Annual Report,* 1898.

floor." A large playhouse, which stood "just above the high water mark, affords the more weakly ones a place of shelter from the sun, and of exposure to the air, where they can lie down or amuse themselves as they may be disposed."[35] The hospital's design and oceanfront location maximized patients' access to sea breezes, fresh air, and ocean water. Structures such as porches and playhouses titrated patients' dose of natural elements.

Even the interior wards reinforced the importance of exposure to the outside environment. Tourists saw that patients stayed in large, open rooms with high ceilings and windows that stretched from the ceiling to the floor. Nurses opened the windows day and night to allow the sea breezes to circulate through the space, thereby removing exhaled air and replacing it with fresh sea breezes. Medical staff only closed the windows when patients changed clothes or during snowstorms and rain showers.[36]

Visitors also learned that health care and healing primarily took place outside. This was true across decades, even after the managers moved the hospital south to escape Atlantic City's encroaching development. As with

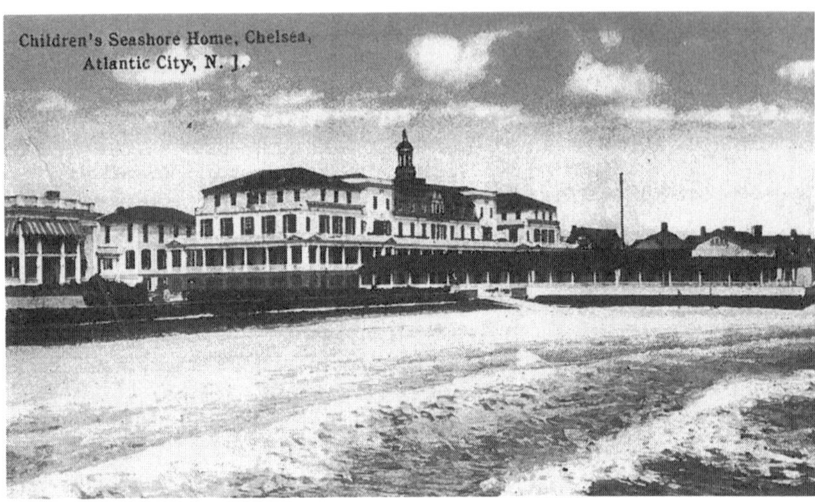

FIGURE 8. Early twentieth-century postcard showing the Children's Seashore House's second permanent structure. Note the similarities in the built environment. As with the first hospital (fig. 7), the main hospital faces the ocean, and mothers' cottages lie along the edges of the property. The overall design highlights the continued importance of the beach location. Published by Virginia Post Card Co. Private collection.

the first hospital, the 1902 structure was a large, white wooden building with a tall main portion flanked by wings. This continuity in design is striking given the changes in medical knowledge and practice.[37] Although physicians and the general public embraced germ theory, the Children's Seashore House expanded and intensified the commitment to environmental therapeutics.

Thus, whether people toured the hospital in the 1870s or in the 1920s, they learned that the seashore was therapeutically advantageous. Patients' activities reinforced the healthfulness of tourists' pastimes, such as swimming and sunbathing. They also saw mothers caring for their children. The Children's Seashore House, like Sea Breeze in New York, built small cottages on the hospital grounds so mothers could stay with their young children. At the Children's Seashore House, two rows of these so-called mothers' cottages lined the north and the south sides of the property, stretching from the main hospital to the ocean's edge.

Looking at the mothers' cottages on the hospital grounds, tourists saw a reflection of the private dwellings in the seaside town. Boosters celebrated Atlantic City's cottage life.[38] The private structures and their relative affordability offered middle-class families the opportunity to vacation in a safe and morally acceptable environment.[39] Largely devoid of the perceived idle or immoral pursuits such as gambling, drinking, and dancing that took place in larger establishments, "cottage cities" enabled families to maintain their domestic routines in a more relaxed, communal setting.[40] Additionally, clusters of cottages provided children with a safe place to wander and play under shared maternal supervision.[41] Visitors likely recognized these arrangements, as they were similar to other seaside tourist neighborhoods. Seeing familiar structures on hospital grounds reinforced the therapeutic association of beach vacations.

Tourists chose to witness marine medication firsthand at hospitals, but some felt less sanguine about sharing the beach with patients. As one of the earliest structures in Atlantic City, the Children's Seashore House sat near the heart of town, close to the train terminal. The popularity of Atlantic City grew, and hotels came to surround the original hospital grounds. By 1894 the physician in charge was lamenting that the hospital was "surrounded by some of the best hotels and cottages on the island, and our humble guests, notwithstanding all our earnest efforts in the direction of neatness and good order, prove to these most unacceptable neighbors."[42] It is unclear whether tourists found the patients "unacceptable" because of the children's physical conditions, class, or race, or some combination thereof. Perhaps the mere presence of bent, broken, and sick pediatric patients reminded otherwise healthy visitors of the urban realities they sought to escape.

Tourists might not want to share the beach with pediatric patients, but the Children's Seashore House remained a defining element of Atlantic City's social scene. In the early twentieth century, the hospital's executive committee invited guests of "as many hotels as could be reached" to attend fundraising teas. William Bennett, the physician in charge of the Children's Seashore House, suggested furthering the work by forming "an Auxiliary Committee of twenty, to be composed as far as practicable of ladies passing the summer in Atlantic City."[43] In 1902, the Mask and Wig, an all-male theater group from the University of Pennsylvania, donated $1,700 from "an entertainment" to the Children's Seashore House.[44]

Atlantic City visitors integrated the Children's Seashore House into the social fabric of everyday life at the beach. Whether visiting the hospital or supporting it through fundraisers, tourists associated the institution with both medical care and entertainment. Outside the hospital grounds, the integration of leisure and pleasure was even more pronounced. Atlantic City's visitors eagerly consumed places and provisions for health. Their actions had lasting consequences.

Bathing for Health or Pleasure?

Up and down the beach, tourists would have seen sights like those they witnessed at seashore hospitals, including ocean bathing. Yet not everyone could enjoy a swim. In 1873, a pamphlet proclaimed that "many unhappy invalids have gazed in sadness upon the joyous throng wrestling with Neptune in the foaming surf, availing themselves of the two-fold healing influences of the saline bath, and the pure life-giving atmosphere, and . . . have prayed that they, too, might be enabled to reap the inestimable benefits almost within their grasp."[45] David C. Spooner understood that visitors' desire to bathe in the sea presented an economic opportunity. He surmised that people would pay if he could bring saltwater bathing to the "timid and the feeble." Spooner then built his "Hot and Cold Salt-Water Bath" business, whose houses resembled large indoor swimming pools. Two "apartments" provided separate spaces for men and women. Each boasted "all the additions and improvements that medical science could devise" and maintained an "elegant style."[46] Most visitors could easily access the baths, located close to hotels.

Patrons suffering from various medical conditions visited, but so too did many healthy tourists. One brochure explained that the baths were "at first intended only for ladies and gentlemen of delicate organization." But after only a year in operation, Spooner's baths were "steadily patronized by the more robust, who find in the quiet retirement and privacy of the baths an agreeable feature."[47] The speed of the transformation is telling. Healthy tourists used the bathhouse despite the institution's original (or at least stated) intention of serving those with medical issues. The bathhouses were popular because they were pleasurable. Not everyone wanted to experience the shock of the cold ocean waters, regardless of whether they physically could.

Atlantic City's guests not only disregarded recommendations about who was meant to use the bathhouses, but they also ignored medical advice when it came to swimming in the ocean. In 1880, Philadelphia-based surgeon John H. Packard published a popular "health-primer" on sea air and sea bathing. The short book included general information for tourists going to the beach. In his introduction Packard argued that "bathing is resorted to for the objects of health, pleasure, and cleanliness" but clarified that sea bathing should be used for health and enjoyment.[48] Packard openly accepted that pleasure was an important aspect of sea bathing. He was vexed, however, that tourists did not understand the potential danger of ocean baths if practiced incorrectly. Packard warned readers that "persons suffering from acute disease in any form ought to abstain from sea-bathing, unless with the express sanction of a competent physician; and the same may be said with regard to all who are laboring under organic affections, whether of the brain, heart, lungs, liver, or kidneys."[49]

Packard offered specific advice on sea bathing for the public. He described how long to bathe and how to best enter the ocean ("walk or run rapidly into the water").[50] He also differentiated floating ("a very pleasant form of bathing") from swimming.[51] Readers learned when to bathe and when not to take the waters, as well as the ideal frequency of sea bathing. Packard also cautioned readers to get out of the water before becoming chilled. In a statement reminiscent of French physician André Brochard's exposition on marine medication, Packard wrote that exposure to the warm sun followed by submersion into the cold ocean water for too long could cause "headache, nausea, and the other symptoms which are generally associated under the term 'biliousness'" and also explained that internal organs, particularly the "nerve-centres," could become congested, causing suffering.[52] Gradual exposure avoided these issues. Bathers needed to be knowledgeable so they could enjoy the benefits of time in the ocean and avoid negative consequences.

If Packard was concerned, tourists were not. Visitors were either unaware of sea bathing's dangers, or simply failed to heed physicians' advice. After

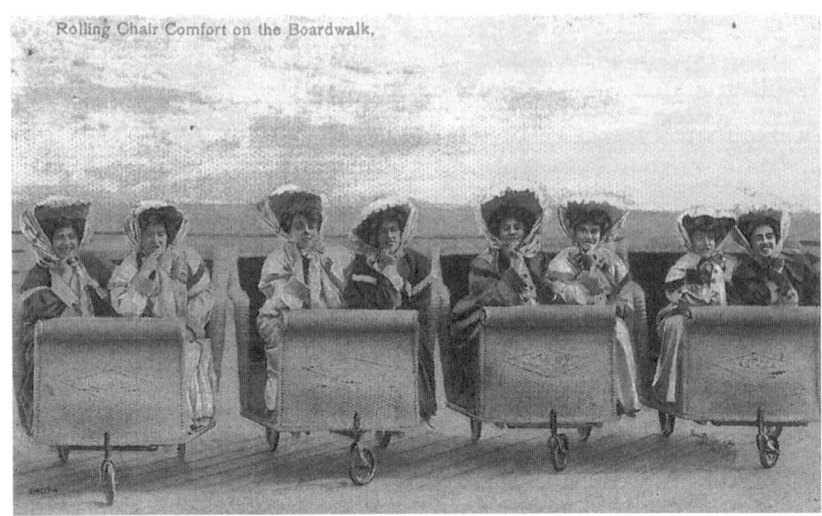

FIGURE 9. "Rolling Chair Comfort on the Boardwalk." This postcard showing women sitting in two-person rolling chairs highlights the fashionable nature of the chairs. Postmarked September 9, 1912, and published by the Post Card Distributing Company, Atlantic City, New Jersey. Author's collection.

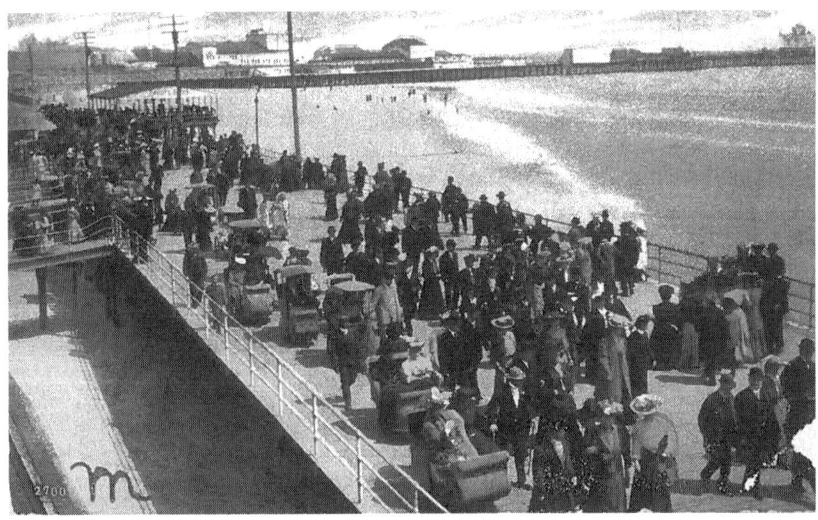

FIGURE 10. "Boardwalk and Young's Pier, Atlantic City, NJ." Rolling chairs line the western edge of the busy boardwalk. Postmarked August 11, 1907, and published by the Souvenir Post Card Company, New York. Author's collection.

rapidly eating, tourists would swim, quickly change clothes, and then visit the amusements that lined the boardwalk and piers. Packard lamented that some of these visitors suffered headaches or stomachaches, although he conceded that "such effects, however, are less frequently observed than might reasonably be supposed."[53] He rationalized this result, suggesting that the change of environment was so beneficial that it outweighed unhygienic and unsafe activities.[54] Even if tourists did not suffer dire consequences by disregarding medical advice, Packard knew they were not receiving the full health benefits from their sea baths.

Spooner's bathhouses and Packard's advice manual offer a glimpse into how tourists simultaneously embraced and transformed one of marine medication's cornerstone practices. Doctors continued to prescribe and recommend tightly controlled sea-bathing regimens, and within hospital walls nurses ensured that patients followed the doctors' orders. On the beach, tourists loosened conventions to the point that they seemed to disappear. The pleasure of bathing indoors or the excitement of plunging into the waves proved more alluring, and less worrisome, than doctors suggested. As tourists took over health care practices and institutions, they shifted cultural associations of these techniques and blended leisure and health.

The Entertaining Transformation of Rolling Chairs

One of the most iconic images of turn-of-the-century Atlantic City depicts rows of rolling chairs lining the boardwalk. Propelled by a "pusher," the wheeled wicker baskets carried between one and three patrons. The chairs symbolized leisure, pleasure, and class and became part of the vanity fair that defined the boardwalk.[55] Rolling chairs even inspired a 1905 song, "Why Don't You Try, or the Rolling Chair Song," about a gentleman suitor and his longing for a curly haired girl named Sue.[56]

Despite their fashionable associations, the chairs were medical devices. Inventors and business owners originally designed wheelchairs for patients who needed assistance moving along the boardwalk. The chairs' transformation underscores the intricate ways in which tourists blended leisure and health at the beach.[57]

Historians debate who introduced rolling chairs to the boardwalk. Some credit Harry Shill, a Philadelphian with mobility issues himself who manufactured transportation devices, including perambulators, go-carts, and "invalid chairs" (wheelchairs).[58] In 1883, Shill decided to cash in on the booming tourism industry in Atlantic City. The town's first boardwalk had been replaced by a wider permanent structure in 1880. The new boardwalk reduced the amount of sand that patrons tracked into hotels and onto trains and made it easier for attendants to push the wheeled devices.

Like Spooner and his bathhouses, Shill initially marketed his rolling chairs to the multitude of so-called disabled and debilitated visitors who sought health at the beach. These medical devices seated only one person and required either a nurse or companion to push them, in what some considered a tiresome venture. Shill later transformed the single-seated chair into a double- and then a triple-occupancy vehicle. This way, the rider could be joined by his or her companions. Patrons could also hire a "pusher," obviating the need for a nurse. In a display of the racial dynamics that defined the time, pushers were most often Black men who had come north seeking employment.[59]

As tourists increasingly used the wheelchairs for pleasure, they transformed the devices. Shill's early versions prioritized function over form and were built with wooden wheels and iron tires.[60] A few years later, his larger chairs became more fashionable with wicker designs, using reeds imported first from Germany and then from the East Indies. New operators, locally called "Barons," quickly joined Shill and established rolling chair stands up and down the boardwalk. Entrepreneurs tweaked Shill's design. J. A. Eveler created "balloon" tires, advertised with the catchy slogan "You ride on air in a [*sic*] Eveler chair."[61] In 1903, Atlantic City resident James B. Howard applied for a US patent for making "new and useful Improvements in Hub-Guards for Wheels" with a specific goal of preventing riders' skirts from becoming caught in rolling chair wheels.[62]

A newspaper article published in March 1903 highlighted the cultural transformation of rolling chairs. In a special to the *New York Times* under the headline "Gorgeous Private Rolling Chairs the Prevailing Fad," the article reported that "the rush to the seashore continues undiminished," despite the season. More noteworthy than the throngs of visitors was the sensation caused by "a beautiful and mysterious woman, who made her appearance on the Boardwalk the other day in a superb private rolling chair." The New York woman and her servants were staying in a rented villa for the season. The landlord refused to divulge the woman's identity, leadings to rumors and speculation. Other tourists gawked in wonder as the woman rolled along the boardwalk in her chair made of "white wood, trimmed with turquoise blue. Its occupant has appeared twice in a costume to match the trimming of the chair, and with a filmy blue veil."[63] This well-to-do visitor was not alone in deploying her chair as a status symbol. Other tourists flaunted private chairs with rubber tires, gilt panels, plate glass windows, family crests, plush upholstery, curtains, and mahogany accents.[64]

It is noteworthy that intrigue, not health-seeking activity, defined the rolling chair in these stories. Their status as cultural symbols continued to shift into the twentieth century. On June 21, 1913, suffragists announced that they would host a roller chair parade in Atlantic City as a prelude to their July 30 demonstration in Washington, DC. Mabel Vernon, a prominent suffragist who organized the famed Washington protests, traveled to Atlantic City, as well as other seaside resorts, to make the argument for votes for women. In Atlantic City the demonstration maintained the culture of seaside resorts by using the chairs to advocate for the cause. Despite the parade's political objectives, organizers attempted to align it with the "vacation spirit" by incorporating banners and flags into the event.[65]

Other women also used rolling chairs to push gender norms.[66] In 1915, the *Washington Post* announced a scandal with this headline: "Seaside Women Smoke." The article dated the trend to a day when "one fair creature in a rolling chair procession blithely and seemingly oblivious of the shocked countenances of sedate boardwalk strollers puffed contentedly away at a cigarette." Over the following days scores of women lounged "languidly against the rattan backs of the moving chairs and indolently enjoy[ed] 'a smoke.'" Protests erupted. As the newspaper reported, "The sight of women smoking in public—so many of them, too—literally staggered visitors with fixed, staid ideas of conventionality." Disturbed tourists complained, but "the police simply winked, shrugged and otherwise demonstrated their helplessness." These were respectable women, beautifully dressed, with "unmistakable marks of breeding." As they rolled along in the chairs, they left behind "wisps of smoke," stares of an indignant public, and people to wonder if this would become something more than a passing fad.[67]

Women smoking in rolling chairs, or fighting for equal voting rights, highlights the change over time. Tourists redefined the chairs in ways that captured headlines for scandals and sightings rather than health restored. Proprietors had no reason to quell the impulse; more users meant more profits.

Clearly these fashionable chairs were no longer medical devices. Yet the uninitiated might be confused by the wheeled chairs that cluttered the boardwalk. Perhaps no one captured this ambiguity more aptly than Arthur Conan Doyle, author of the Sherlock Holmes series. When Doyle first arrived in Atlantic City in the 1930s, he saw the rows of "huge invalid chairs" and thought that only convalescents populated the seaside resort. He quickly discovered his mistake and came to appreciate the joys of riding in rolling chairs. Although brief, Doyle's stay in Atlantic City provided him with enough time to reengineer his original impression.[68] By 1930, the cultural pendulum had swung so far that even a wheelchair could change into a form of entertainment.

AS EARLY AS 1887, Atlantic City used the tagline "For Health and Pleasure" to entice tourists to visit the seaside town.[69] Time changed associations and practices, but tourists and the tourism industry still promoted the beach as a therapeutic environment. In 1918, Atlantic City booster Earle Ovington released a pamphlet encouraging visitors to come to Atlantic City, claiming, "There's robust health awaiting you in Atlantic City. You have but to come here for a while to prove the truth of this statement."[70] Ovington confided that he initially felt skeptical of sweeping claims regarding the therapeutic benefits of the seashore. He became convinced only after experiencing the healthfulness of the beach firsthand.

Ovington championed Atlantic City's therapeutic components. He boasted that the city offered "three of the greatest health-giving elements known to science; sunshine, ozone and recreation." He heralded the town's sunlight with its "vitalizing rays in their fullest intensity," its purifying ozone in the atmosphere, and its recreational opportunities. He explained that Atlantic

City's attractions prevented visitors from worrying about work or responsibilities. The freedom from concerns allowed sunlight and ozone to work their health-giving magic.[71]

Ovington also tied Atlantic City's benefits to older travel prescriptions: "When you go to your physician and tell him your brain is full of cobwebs, or your liver is misbehaving itself, what does he say in nine cases out of ten? 'Take a sea voyage if you can spare the time.'" Of course, Ovington recognized, not many could afford such a trip. Atlantic City, he argued, provided patients an attractive, accessible alternative with its five-mile boardwalk. Walking along the promenade, or being rolled in one of the popular wheeled chairs, afforded visitors "the same vitalizing, salt-laden air, and oceanward you have the same tumbling waves stretching as far as the eye can see." However, when they bored of such vistas, tourists could simply turn around and avail themselves of the restaurants, shops, and amusements that lined the other side of the boardwalk. Ovington explained that time on the boardwalk had the benefits of ocean travel, "minus the seasickness and inconveniences."[72]

But Ovington also recognized that popular perceptions had changed. When he wrote on behalf of Atlantic City, he promoted tourism and emphasized recreation alongside the therapeutic effects of sun and sea air. Indeed, for medical practitioners and the general public, health required access to recreation as well as fresh air and sunlight. In the twentieth century, the seashore remained a healthful escape from urban life. Physicians and the public understood that the psychological benefits of pleasure and leisure at the beach equaled the health benefits the physical environment provided.

In many ways the momentum toward pleasure and away from health seems predictable, medically and culturally. It fits within the wider belief system that defined the seaside as the antithesis to the city. Cities were places of work, responsibility, and toil. Thus, when tourists went to the seashore, they found health but discovered leisure and pleasure as well. Over the decades entertainment gathered steam at America's seaside resorts. Atlantic City attracted folks who wanted to watch the first Miss America pageant, witness the diving horses, take in a boxing match, or be entertained by the Rat Pack. Farther north, Coney Island offered tourists marvels and amusements with carnival-type rides and performances.[73]

Although transformational, the changes to the seascape did not require that tourists reject the idea that the seaside instilled health. But like Doyle's experience with the rolling chairs, the association with health was fleeting, remote, and increasingly hard to see. As tourists consumed medical practices and disregarded physicians' advice, they shifted popular perceptions of the beach away from health.

In time, even the once popular Children's Seashore House moved to the edge of town and hosted fewer guests. Some famous actors, musicians, and the circus still came. However, visitors went to entertain the children, not to witness marine medication. These changes are symbolic of larger cultural shifts. By 1930, Pitney's grand health resort had become a place that people popularized as a landscape of leisure, entertainment, and recreation. Americans did not reject the seashore as a therapeutic landscape but instead transformed it through their consumption of marine medication's practices and technologies.

FOUR HOW WORKING-CLASS MOTHERS SHAPED THE SHORE

WORKING-CLASS MOTHERS established the American public's notion of the northeastern seaboard as a space of health and leisure. In the summertime they packed their bags, gathered their children, and temporarily escaped the difficulties of urban life. They sought relief from stifling and sickening summertime temperatures. Their experiences contributed to the ongoing popularity of beach vacations, and their presence reinforced beliefs that the seashore was a healthy space for families from a wide range of financial backgrounds.

Retracing women's footsteps highlights their impact on the seashore and Americans' perceptions of it. In Philadelphia, mothers boarded trains with their children and traveled to Atlantic City, New Jersey. As the trains chugged along their tracks, families would have looked out their windows and watched the scenery change during the two-hour trip. Departing from Philadelphia, they crossed the Delaware River, traveled through the city of Camden, New Jersey, before passing through small Quaker towns such as Haddonfield, New Jersey. They traversed expanses of farmland and pine forest before finally arriving at the shore.

Reaching Atlantic City, working-class mothers and children made their way to cottage lodgings. Unlike more well-to-do women, they did not arrive at a privately owned or rented abode. Rather, many families checked into cottages on the grounds of the Children's Seashore House. Walking toward the hospital, they would have first seen a three-story white building with a flag whipping in the breeze. Inside the main hospital, a nurse registered each family, recording such information as the patients' names, ages, addresses, and the children's diagnoses.

Once signed in, mothers exited the back of the hospital and encountered a grand sight. The ocean sparkled just a couple hundred yards in front of them.[1] An expanse of beach operated like a gigantic sand garden for children. Two rows of cottages stretched along the southern and northern property lines, extending from the main hospital building toward the ocean, creating a haven for children to lounge, dig, and play.

Having surveyed the scene, mothers trekked across the beachfront property, heels sinking into the sand as they walked. Finding their designated cottage, mothers aided young children as they climbed the steps to the porch of the one-room structure. They opened the door to discover a room filled with sunlight and sea breezes that swirled through two large windows on either side of the cottage's front door and another that stretched across the back wall. Perusing the interior, mothers found a double-sized iron bed with a woven wire mattress, a table with chairs, a rocking chair, and a crib. A second porch flanked the back of the unit and provided additional shade. There was even a bell that connected the cottage to the main building, allowing mothers to summon a nurse.[2]

Women went to great lengths to gain admission to these so-called mothers' cottages. Some trudged miles through the city, children in tow, to reach a referring physician, hoping they would receive an admissions slip. If the physician approved, mothers received a ticket and paid from one to three dollars a week for room and board.[3] The hospital covered the fee for those who were too poor to pay, and railroad companies assisted families by reducing train fares. Philadelphia mothers were not alone in their experiences. Women from New York City made similar trips to Coney Island's health homes, run by children's aid societies, as well as to cottages operated by the Association for Improving the Condition of the Poor at Sea Breeze Hospital.[4]

Working-class mothers' annual summertime pilgrimages disrupt what we think we know about American tourism. Historians have documented the rise of travel among upper- and middle-classes families in the nineteenth century and into the twentieth.[5] Working-class tourists, and mothers and children especially, are notably absent from most accounts.[6] Looking at the cottages at seaside hospitals makes clear that working-class families, and women in particular, were notable in their presence at the beach. Analyzing mothers' practices at seashore institutions provides new insights into how working-class women contributed to cultural associations about the beach as a landscape of health and leisure.[7]

It makes sense that mothers, regardless of social class, would want to go to the shore. We know these women understood that their urban environments and long hours of work drained their bodies of health and vigor.[8] They witnessed the same effects in their children. It follows that they would take advantage of the opportunity to escape the hot, congested city and seek relief at the beach. As detailed in chapter 1, mothers adopted the practice of seeking health by frequenting parks, playgrounds, and institutions that offered temporary trips outside the city. Traveling to the seashore was an extension of these practices.[9]

As working-class women traveled between their urban homes and the beach, they influenced cultural practices and attitudes, effectively expanding gender boundaries and influencing pleasure pursuits.[10] The women enjoyed the communal experiences at hospitals, mirroring other seaside communities such as the cottages of Wesleyan Grove on Martha's Vineyard.[11] Some women traveled with friends, neighbors, or family members, while others brought babysitters. Even those who traveled alone benefited from the camaraderie of other mothers and assistance from the nursing staff. When women stayed at institutions like the Children's Seashore House, they did not have to prepare or clean up after meals, work a job, or try to protect their children from urban dangers. Instead, they could relax while watching their children play in the relative comfort of the beach under the watchful gaze of others.

Analyzing mothers' experiences at places like the Children's Seashore House cottages restores working-class women's place in the historical record as actors who transformed ideas about the seashore, bodies, and health. This chapter expands our historical framing by situating working-class mothers as actors who shaped and promoted geographies of health and who constructed the beach as a landscape that could both cure kids and provide respite for women. We will see that mothers who sought admission to hospital cottages acted as tourists and consumers, much like their middle- and upper-class counterparts. They made demands, expected a degree of autonomy, and sought repose. When they returned to the city, they reported their experiences to friends and family and encouraged others to make a similar trip.

Working-class women spread knowledge of America's seashore as a place where families of almost any means could find health, leisure, and reprieve from the difficulties that defined urban life.

The City's Push

The push to leave the city matched the pull of the sea. In August 1881, the *Daily Graphic*, a New York City newspaper, ran a drawing ironically labeled "Summer Resorts of the Poor."[12] It showed a family sitting on a rooftop in the city. An exhausted and run-down mother holds an infant on her lap, as her glum-looking husband sits beside her. Two girls sleep beneath the woman's legs. In the background, a young boy uses a large shovel to scoop dirt into a pail, while another child sits with his hand cocked, ready to throw something at the sleeping girls. The caption reads: "*Mother*: 'Tom, Stop throwing pebbles at your sisters. Let the poor things sleep!' *Tom* (*sadly*)—'Well, Mother, this is all of the sea-shore we can have, we might have a little fun with it.'"[13] Given the squalid surroundings and her forlorn expression, one can imagine that mothers like Tom's would have eagerly swapped their urban rooftops for cottages overlooking the Atlantic Ocean.

To understand why working-class mothers sought admission to seaside hospital cottages, it helps to understand the pressures, responsibilities, and environments they wanted to escape. As documented in chapter 1, mothers confronted ceaseless domestic and child-care duties. Urban working-class families' environmental and familial circumstances made such tasks particularly difficult. Feeding children presented one challenge. Affording nutritious food was an issue, and adults fretted about the weak, wan, and skinny youths who roamed the city streets. Accessing safe dairy milk was another problem, especially for families with infants. Mothers knew that babies were especially vulnerable to malnourishment and the effects of impure milk, and infant mortality rates cast light on just how many babies died before reaching their first birthdays.[14]

The urban milk supply contributed to this issue. In the mid-nineteenth century, milk sellers adulterated their supplies to increase their profits. Some farmers fed their cows "slop" by-product from distilleries. These cows, and their milk, were nutritionally depleted. In order to mask the poor quality, producers added substances such as starch, plaster of Paris, chalk, flour, and eggs to approximate the color and consistency of milk produced by healthy cows. Unsuspecting mothers purchased this milk for their infants.[15] Public officials and newspapers decried the health effects caused by tainted, spoiled, and skimmed milk. They demanded legislation to regulate quality and distribution and argued that pure milk could reduce infant mortality by up to 25 percent. New York successfully outlawed "swill milk" in the mid-nineteenth century. By the end of the century many cities had milk dispensaries that supplied urban mothers with pure milk and instructions for handling and storage.[16]

In addition to feeding responsibilities, mothers also had to keep clean and healthy homes.[17] This was an arduous task for working-class mothers. Keeping residences free of dirt, grime, and offensive smells represented a herculean responsibility. They would have spent countless hours sweeping, washing, and scrubbing to combat smells, all to little avail.

Fighting filth was always difficult, and the widespread lack of plumbing made the situation even worse. In 1890, only 24 percent of US homes had running water. By 1911, the situation had improved little. While more houses had access to water, they often contained only a single faucet in the kitchen or a hydrant in the yard. Washing was particularly laborious. Women lugged buckets of water to clean woodwork, floors, and dishes, and they especially lamented laundry day. For mothers with young children, washing diapers and clothes was an endless cycle.[18]

In the quest for cleanliness, working-class families faced additional challenges of limited financial resources, which resulted in large families living in small dwellings. Journalist and social and environmental reformer Jacob Riis published photographs that documented these hardships in his book *How the Other Half Lives*. His photographs cast light into the dark corners of New York's working-class homes, vividly depicting the difficulties families faced.[19] Readers could witness firsthand the crowded confines of urban slums. Housing in the poorest communities lacked the most basic elements for ensuring health. In New York, tenement apartments sometimes did not have windows, which made ventilation and sunlight sparse and resulted in stifling heat and suffocating smells. In other cities, such as Philadelphia, homes might have more space, but inadequate drainage created breeding grounds for disease. Working-class mothers also lacked the time and money necessary for the air-purifying practices of their wealthier counterparts.[20]

Despite the obvious hardships, government officials, settlement workers, and child welfare advocates pressed mothers to do more to create environments that protected their children's health and well-being. In 1913, officials from the US Children's Bureau announced that mothers needed to learn how to combat infant mortality by attending to their home environment *and* the milk they fed their babies. Officials still stressed the importance of pure milk but warned that "it is useless to send pure, clean milk into a dirty home to be handled by an ignorant, dirty mother or older child." They advanced maternal education campaigns so mothers could learn "the necessity of cleanliness" and "the deadliness of dirt," particularly "where the baby's food is concerned."[21]

Imagine standing alongside a young working-class mother who was the subject of these campaigns, such as the three little Donoghys' mother in chapter 1. It's the end of the day, and she has been at work, perhaps washing clothes. The evening is hot, and garments cling to bodies. You look around the mother's apartment that is in one of the city's most densely inhabited neighborhoods. There are no windows to open, just a door to a dark hallway. You see her family members and maybe a tenant or two nestled wherever they can find space. Their bodies are marked by a day of working or playing outside in the street. The absurdity of gleaming floors and tidy rooms, full plates and contented bellies, and ruddy cheeks filling out dirt-free faces is obvious. It is not hard to believe the mother would want to escape.

The Ocean's Pull

Pediatric seashore hospitals and health homes gave urban mothers a place to breathe, literally and figuratively. At the Children's Seashore House, mothers stayed in cottages that architects had designed with ventilation, drainage, and sunlight in mind.[22] While women had to keep the residence clean during their stay, nurses and staff assisted with many of the other tasks of motherhood. Hospital staff prepared and served meals and washed the dishes. The main hospital building had indoor plumbing, with hot and cold water.[23] Nurses and mothers shared child-care responsibilities, watching children play and tending to their well-being.

Mothers clamored for admission. In 1885, one of the Children's Seashore House's Philadelphia-based "examining physicians" assessed nearly six hundred mothers and children every summer to determine their suitability for admission. Many women, he wrote, walked to his office with a "sick babe, and frequently one or two little children, a mile or two, through the heat of July and August," just for the chance of going to the seaside hospital.[24] In 1899, Children's Seashore House head physician William Bennett told supporters that the entity had grown beyond what people had imagined at its founding. That year, nineteen urban hospitals and institutions requested admission on behalf of children. Thousands of mothers sought admission for themselves and their children as well. The hospital had to deny hundreds for lack of space.[25]

In Philadelphia, working-class mothers sought admission to the seaside facility's cottages beginning in 1875, when they first opened. In the early decades, many mothers brought critically ill infants for what they hoped would be lifesaving care. In 1875, thirteen of the sixteen babies had "some form of summer Diarrhea." The other three had various conditions, including bronchitis, debility, and marasmus, an extreme form of malnutrition that resulted in low weight.[26] The medical staff and mothers knew that infantile diarrhea claimed the lives of thousands of babies every summer. Time at the beach seemed to breathe life back into the sick babes, with many improving and others recovering entirely.

During the summer of 1881, Dr. Bennett acknowledged both the popularity of the cottages and women's belief in the benefits of marine medication. Although the Children's Seashore House could accommodate one hundred mothers each season, Bennett reported that, on one hand, he repeatedly had to "listen to the entreaties of mothers asking to be allowed to stay until their infants were beyond the danger of relapse; and on the other to receive by letter and telegram appeals from parents or friends for the immediate admission of children who had been long waiting for vacancies and whose only hope seemed to be prompt removal from the city."[27] The prospects of lifesaving care inspired urban mothers to seek admission for their families and to clamor to stay once admitted.

Some mothers were so desperate to access care that they bypassed admissions procedures and went straight to the hospital. In the summer of 1886, two local women appealed to the Children's Seashore House staff. Both had babies in dire need of medical attention. One mother, a servant for a family in Atlantic City, brought her sick child directly to the hospital, where she requested admission. The second woman waited outside the hospital, and the medical staff found the "unhappy mother, wandering helpless, unhoused and unfed, on the board-walk in front of the institution." That mother cradled her dying baby in her arms. Nurses welcomed both mothers and their babies into the hospital despite knowing that the infants were "beyond mortal succor." The staff was correct, and both babies died. While it was not the outcome anyone hoped, the staff admitted the mothers so that their babies' "last hours might be made more comfortable."[28] Moreover, the physician in charge argued that these two cases indicated "the great usefulness of the House" as "the poor mothers feel that the House was a refuge for them in their distress."[29] Even accounting for the promotional nature of the doctor's assertions, these stories frame mothers as active agents who sought and appreciated the care at seashore hospitals.

Other sources support the conclusion that women embraced seashore hospitals as lifesaving resources. Helen Stainthorpe, a mother who stayed at the Children's Seashore House, wrote to the *Philadelphia Inquirer* in 1901.[30] Stainthorpe described herself as a poor woman and a coal miner's wife. She had immigrated to Wilkes-Barre, Pennsylvania, an industrial town located 120 miles northwest of Philadelphia.[31] Stainthorpe recounted reading an article in the *Philadelphia Inquirer* about the Children's Seashore House that inspired her to seek help for her child. Her three-year-old daughter Amy had been sick for more than two years. Stainthorpe described Amy as being "not as big as some children at six months. Her legs are tiny and she cannot walk. The doctors say she has rickets. We have done everything we could for her. When I read in your paper about the Children's Seashore House I wished my little girl could go there, and so I wrote to ask them about it and I got a letter back to tell me to come and bring the three children, and I went by an excursion on the 7th of August."[32] Stainthorpe brought Amy and her two other daughters to the hospital by the sea. The doctors confirmed Amy's diagnosis of rickets and noted her sisters were both "delicate." The physician admitted the family into one of the mothers' cottages. All of the children "improved" over the course of their stay.[33]

The family remained at the Seashore House for eleven days. Eventually it was time for them to leave, but despite her progress, Amy's condition warranted additional time at the beach. The medical staff transferred the child to the main hospital building, where she stayed with other patients until her grandmother came in September. The grandmother and granddaughter moved back into one of the cottages and stayed there for an additional five days until the hospital closed for the season.[34] At the end of the summer, Amy went to St. Christopher's Hospital in Philadelphia, the hospital's winter annex.

In her letter to the editor, Stainthorpe expressed confidence that Amy would recover and conveyed her appreciation for the staff. She wrote, "Everyone treated me so well," and she specifically acknowledged Miss Jeffrey, the "lady superintendent," for her kindness.[35] Concluding her letter, Stainthorpe proclaimed that "if she [Amy] gets well, as I believe she will, I shall bless the day I read of it in your paper."[36]

Helen Stainthorpe's experience cannot stand in for every mother who took advantage of the cottages. It does, however, illustrate several important elements of working-class mothers' mind-sets and their contributions to ongoing cultural conversations and medical beliefs. Stainthorpe's ready embrace of the Children's Seashore House suggests that she shared medical professionals' vision of the beach's therapeutic potential. She had sought medical care within her industrial city to no avail. Stainthorpe was driven to access better medical care for her ailing daughter, but no one compelled her to go to the seaside hospital or to leave Amy there. Stainthorpe's request for admission indicates that ultimately the decision to send a child to the Children's Seashore House often lay with women, not their husbands or physicians. It made sense to mothers, as it did to many others, that the seashore provided benefits that exceeded those of urban institutions and home-based care. Stainthorpe's decision to allow Amy to stay for additional treatment highlights the strength of this belief, as well as her comfort with the level of care her child would receive.

When working-class mothers like Stainthorpe embraced seaside institutions, they reinforced medical beliefs about the curative potential of the beach.

Mothers and children continued to trek from their urban homes to seaside hospitals well into the twentieth century, and the hospital continued to promote the curative effects of a stay by the sea. In 1908, the Children's Seashore House Board of Managers reported that the hospitals had admitted 177 babies with "diseases which usually make up the summer mortality." They celebrated that 170 of these babies returned home to their families and were still alive. Among the other 7, 2 died during their stay at the hospital and another 5 or 6 died after being discharged. The survival rate of approximately 96 percent was remarkable when the best urban hospitals recorded mortality rates that approached 50 percent.[37] Such results strengthened the association that the seashore could cure sick children.

Mothers' firsthand accounts further supported the knowledge that the beach benefited families of all economic backgrounds. When mothers brought babies and children to seaside hospitals and health homes, they witnessed their children's health improve. They also discovered that they could access a bit of relief for themselves.

Seeking Leisure in a Hospital

Mothers still flocked to seaside hospitals in the twentieth century, but their motivation for seeking admission began to shift from health to relaxation. By this time improvements in sanitation, nutrition, and the milk supply had reduced childhood death and disease. Infant mortality rates in cities such as Philadelphia and New York fell in the first two decades of the twentieth century.[38] Correspondingly, seaside hospitals catered to fewer infants suffering from diarrheal diseases, which created space in the cottages for children with a wider range of ailments.

By the 1910s, the patient population at seaside hospitals had changed, reflecting these shifts. Many mothers brought children who were "well" or suffered from a mild, non-life-threatening ailment. The admissions records from 1916 describe a mother named Nellie Oates who went with her three children to the Children's Seashore House; each child suffered a range of conditions, from indigestion to eczema.[39] None had life-threatening ailments like the babies admitted in the 1870s and 1880s. Oates returned with her children for five more summers, even when her children were perfectly healthy. In 1920, their last year to stay at the Children's Seashore House, the Oates children were like most of the patients who stayed in the cottages at this time: they came and left the institution in a healthy state.

Mothers bringing healthy children to a hospital defies logic, unless they sought something other than health care. Their practices suggest that women sought a vacation and a break from urban life. The conclusion that they viewed seaside hospitals differently from other institutions is supported by the fact that women and caregivers often rejected city-based hospitalization for themselves and their children. Particularly before 1900, Americans viewed hospitals as institutions of last resort; only destitute and friendless patients used them. As pediatric hospitals opened in cities, parents shunned them as well. Institutional policies curtailed or prevented parental visits, and mothers and fathers lamented their inability to visit and comfort their sick children.[40] With the rise of scientific medicine, parents also feared their children becoming the objects of dangerous medical experiments.[41] Health care remained largely within homes at the behest of mothers.

The fact that mothers advocated for admission to seaside hospitals when they scorned urban institutions indicates they viewed seaside cottages differently. Mothers' actions and experiences suggest that they—like wealthier women—sought the seashore as a space of relative leisure. Journalists' reports support the conclusion that mothers went with their children to seashore hospitals to escape the burdens of urban life.[42] One mother told a reporter that the Seaside Hospital in New York "is the only place this side of Heaven that a poor woman doesn't have to work," while another concurred, exclaiming that if "Heaven is anything like the Seaside Hospital, I don't care how soon I get there."[43] With fewer responsibilities or worries, as well as access to a healthy environment, working-class mothers discovered that the seashore was a space of relaxation relative to their urban lives. In this way they achieved some of the repose that psychologists and reformers defined as important for women.[44]

Women shared with their urban friends and family, as well as doctors, nurses, and social workers, details about their experiences at the beach. In 1899, William Bennett of the Children's Seashore House celebrated that "knowledge of the great benefits which many such children derive from a stay at the seashore has gradually found its way not only into the homes of the poor, but also into the hospitals themselves."[45] Working-class mothers spread knowledge of seaside hospitals' benefits and encouraged others to take advantage of the resource. Women thus cultivated vernacular pathways of knowledge and promoted the seashore as an environment of health and leisure where they belonged.

In the early twentieth century, urban mothers strengthened the association of the seashore with leisure by traveling with families, friends, and neighbors to seaside hospitals. These institutions' infrastructure maintained family and caregiving networks. Traveling with loved ones likely alleviated mothers' fear of, and anguish at, being separated from their children. Organizations that served urban working-class families supported the practices of keeping kin together. The Starr Centre Association, a social organization located in South Philadelphia, referred four families to the Children's Seashore House, and the families stayed at the hospital the same week.[46] Two of these mothers, Rose and Sabatina Frugoli, were likely sisters-in-law, making their children cousins. Like many other families, they returned together during a subsequent summer, staying with their children for a week.[47]

Historical records also suggest that mothers recommended the Children's Seashore cottages to their friends. In July 1919, the Stockman family stayed in one of the mothers' cottages for nine days. None of the children was sick at admission or discharge.[48] It must have been a pleasant, even vacation-like experience; records hint that Stockman recommended time at the cottages to her friends after she returned to her home on Tree Street in South Philadelphia.[49] Later in the summer, her neighbor Mrs. Steer went to the Children's Seashore House for six days with her three children, ages one, four, and six.[50] The following July, the Steer and Stockman families returned to the cottages there. Not only did they travel together with healthy children in tow, but they also brought along another neighborhood family.[51]

Between 1918 and 1923, over 120 families came to the seashore hospital with neighbors.[52] The practice of traveling to the beach with family and friends seems strikingly familiar, even today. As many parents know, having playmates for children often lessens the burden of travel. The preference for traveling with others bolsters the idea that urban, working-class mothers went to the seashore for relief from some of duties of motherhood. Going to the hospital with acquaintances provided mothers with camaraderie and assistance with children.

Some mothers also brought children who were close in age to their own, perhaps to serve as playmates.[53] This arrangement would have been enjoyable for the children, while also alleviating some responsibilities for the mothers who remained in the city. Mothers additionally lightened their own caregiving responsibilities by having an additional pair of hands during their stay in the cottages. Girls between the ages of ten and fourteen went with families other than their own, acting as babysitters or "little mothers."[54] Institutions capitalized on the girls' presence and taught them child-rearing techniques. Although the girls shouldered responsibilities, they had the support of nurses and the benefits of providing child care on the beach instead of on city streets.

Mothers' practices of bringing a "little mother" and traveling with friends shows that women recognized the work involved in temporarily relocating their families. While the Children's Seashore House provided relief from domestic duties such as cooking, mothers still had to oversee their children. The institutions also demanded that women maintain their cottages' cleanliness. Mothers had to keep their cottage floors swept, an unenviable task given children's sandy feet after a day on the beach. Indeed, Atlantic City installed its famous boardwalk in response to complaints from hotels and railroad companies about all the sand that patrons tracked indoors.

Despite some domestic tasks, the Children's Seashore cottages provided a landing spot for working-class mothers who felt the pull to spend time at the beach with their children. From the mothers' point of view, time at the cottages allowed them to escape the city while maintaining ties to their urban communities. During their stay, they enjoyed the company of other women and assistance with the daily tasks and chores incumbent to everyday life in the city. The women who traveled to seaside hospital homes and cottages affirmed that the beach was a place their families belonged, in pursuit of children's health and mothers' leisure.

Negotiating Cottage Responsibilities

Seaside hospitals countered prevailing institutional trends by keeping families and friends together. Tending to families in private cottages created far more work for the nurses and staff and reflected health care practices often reserved for wealthy patrons.[55] The system, however, aligned with physicians' conceptualization of the seashore as a site of health care. While urban-based practitioners increasingly turned toward the laboratory and its pathogenic view of disease, clinicians at seaside hospitals maintained their dedication to environmental interventions to promote physical and mental well-being. Marine medication practitioners believed the cottages could provide both curative and preventive health benefits.

Not all women appreciated their time at the hospital-based cottages, and medical professionals did not uniformly embrace every mother. Tensions could arise when medical providers' health care objectives conflicted with mothers' wishes. In the nineteenth century, disagreements occurred when some women did not meet the standards of decorum required by the institution. By the twentieth century, medical professionals were expressing frustrations when women refused to comply with rules.

Issues arose when some mothers took advantage of the nursing staff and relied on them as babysitters. In 1924, a Mrs. Edwards brought her five children to the hospital for twelve days. While four of the children were admitted as being "well," Margaret, the second eldest, suffered from tuberculosis of the hip. During their stay, the nurse noted that the mother was "undesirable" because she "always insists on leaving children in Wards," instead of watching the children herself.[56] This practice vexed the nurse, who viewed Edwards as shirking her responsibilities. Edwards's actions suggest that she felt, and enacted, a degree of agency despite being a patient. She ceded her children's care to the hospital staff, earning herself a reprieve from her maternal duties.

Other women's experiences bolster the conclusion that mothers exerted a degree of autonomy during cottage stays. Dr. Bennett had advocated that the staff maintain a day care intended "to relieve each mother of the care of her children a short time each day that she may get a little needed rest and receive at our hands some instruction in the care of her children and her home."[57] In the summer of 1925, four mothers rejected this recommendation. The nurse recorded that one mother "stayed 2 days. Would not take child to nursery." The other three mothers similarly "refused" to place their children and left the hospital before their allotted time had elapsed.[58] While women's power may not have been on par with that of the medical staff, they voted with their feet and left.

Such actions demonstrate that some mothers resented what they perceived as intrusion into their leisure and their autonomy in rearing children. Nurses complained that some mothers were "undesirable," "dirty," and "annoying" and condemned women who did not adequately clean the cottages.[59] In August 1923, a Children's Seashore House nurse wrote that one mother who was admitted with her two "well" children was problematic because she "used bed pillows in baby coach."[60] Considering this from the perspective of the mothers, women were making their stay at the beach more comfortable and relaxing by rejecting rules and chores and by providing comfort for their children.

Pejorative comments from health care staff are unsurprising. Like many other institutions that cared for working-class families, the Children's Seashore House wanted to reach the so-called worthy poor.[61] Bennett even advocated screening mothers before admission to attract only the "most deserving women."[62] By the 1900s, the hospital was employing a "social visitor," a Miss Bartley, whose job included visiting families in their homes to determine their need and respectability.[63]

Even with these safeguards in place, some mothers used the facility to meet their own ends rather than the goals of the hospital's administrators and its board. Nurses became frustrated by mothers who consumed the institution's resources when they believed those mothers could afford to go elsewhere. One part of the social visitor's job was to ensure that "abuses . . . by the well-to-do" did not occur in the form of families falsely claiming poverty.[64] She found that most but not all families met the hospital's standards. Some mothers slipped through the cracks across the decades. In July 1924, the cottage nurse wrote that Harriet M., a mother who was admitted with one child, was "entirely too prosperous."[65] In June 1925, a nurse wrote up another mother for asking for free admission despite being "well dressed" and having "money to lend."[66]

In addition to ensuring that their resources went to the neediest families, the hospital staff also upheld its mission to serve patients "without regard to creed, color, or nationality."[67] When nurses recorded mothers' unsanitary practices, they did not map them onto racialized lines as we might expect. Rather, nurses were protective of the Black families who came. In 1926, nurses made record of a group of siblings who were "prejudiced against colored folks," likely as a warning against admitting the family in the future.[68] This aligns with racial integration at other pediatric institutions and even urban swimming pools at the time.[69] Moreover, specific behaviors, rather than race or immigration status, dictated when conflicts arose between patients and providers. Caring for the urban masses mattered more to the physicians and nurses than the color of patients' skin or the countries from which they came.[70]

Understanding hospital rules tells us how medical professionals understood the benefits of their work, as well as what mothers' expectations may have been. Mothers knew they were staying at a hospital and therefore should have anticipated that policies such as maintaining a "sanitary" space would be enforced.[71] Yet some mothers were unwilling to adhere to these regulations, suggesting that too much cleaning or child care interfered with their respite from their responsibilities at home.

In many ways working-class mothers behaved like other tourists who sought seaside vacations. They acted like consumers. Several patients complained about the food, and one family left early because of it.[72] Another mother demanded to be moved from her assigned cottage, claiming an insect infestation. While it is unclear if the staff acquiesced, the mother enjoyed her experience enough to request an extension. When she learned that her request was denied, the woman threatened to report the cottages' "filthy conditions" to the managers.[73] Complaining about the food and lodging implies that working-class women saw the mothers' cottages as a service they paid for, more than a medical interaction that complied with traditional patient-provider roles.

What is most striking, however, is how seldom conflicts arose. Nurses made sparse annotations in the cottages' admissions records, and not all comments were negative. The relative lack of marginalia, and specifically negative notes, suggests that practitioners' and mothers' goals often aligned. If mothers sought leisure, hospitals were willing to provide it. Physicians and the middle class had embraced vacations to replenish the energy that cities drained. This commonality dovetailed with scientists' messages about the importance of rest for women. Psychologists promoted programs of relaxation to restore health and well-being. William James preached the "gospel of relaxation," while Annie Payson Call wrote *Power through Repose*, wherein she encouraged women to train their nerves to preserve and recuperate vital energy.[74]

Working-class mothers may not have been the intended audience, but spaces like seaside hospital cottages allowed them temporary liberation from some domestic duties. A stay at the cottages reinforced the association that the beach was a site for health and leisure.

One important difference is that unlike middle-class families, who stayed in private homes or hotels while visiting the beach, working-class mothers stayed at seashore hospitals and could not disaggregate their experiences from therapeutic influences. Nevertheless, very few mothers left the hospital before their scheduled discharge, and others returned with friends and neighbors, some for multiple summers. Inferring beliefs from actions tells us that mothers viewed seaside cottages, whether located within or beyond a hospital's bounds, as a vacation destination.

WORKING-CLASS MOTHERS promoted cultural practices that established the seashore as a therapeutic landscape and a place where urban families could access leisure. When mothers brought sick children to the seaside cottages, they reinforced prevailing ideas that the beach could cure. Like Helen Stainthorpe, these women shared their experiences that sick children could heal and recover at the beach. When they returned home, they spread this knowledge throughout their urban communities, among family and friends. Largely in concert with the medical staff, mothers rejected the standard form of institutional, custodial care.

Working-class women also embraced the beach because it provided leisure and a break from everyday responsibilities. When mothers brought healthy children to seashore hospitals, they appropriated and shifted associations with these organizations, from seeing them as health care institutions to regarding them as sites of tourism. They actively negotiated their experiences by traveling with companions, rejecting rules, and embracing a break from urban responsibilities. In these ways working-class mothers behaved much like the tourists who transformed rolling chairs and bathhouses from medical technologies into pleasurable pursuits.

Yet working-class mothers who stayed at hospital cottages could not extricate themselves from the medical infrastructure of their seaside retreats. Even if they sought pleasure and leisure, many found it in the shadow of the hospital in which they stayed. Regardless, women established and maintained the beach as a popular vacation destination for urban American families.

FIVE PEDIATRIC PATIENTS AT THE BEACH

ALONGSIDE MOTHERS AND TOURISTS, children also shaped life at the beach. From the earliest years of seaside tourism, they occupied the landscape as well as popular images and stories about the seashore. In the late 1860s, when readers first entered the world of *Little Women*, they learned that the March sisters believed that the beach could cure. In the book, Jo sent her younger sister, Beth, to the seashore to recover from scarlet fever. Even "though Beth didn't come home as plump and rosy as could be desired, she was much better."[1] When Beth's condition deteriorated again, Jo sent her back to the beach. Jo hoped that Beth "could live much in the open air, and let the fresh sea breezes blow a little color into her pale cheeks."[2]

Louisa May Alcott was not the only author who sent young characters to the beach. In 1907, young readers could follow *The Bobbsey Twins at the Seashore*, while just over fifteen years later kids could read about *Honey Bunch: Her First Visit to the Seashore*.[3] Both books described youthful experiences of families on vacation.

The seashore continued to appear as a therapeutic landscape in children's literature. In 1922, Margery Williams published *The Velveteen Rabbit*, a tale about a stuffed animal that comforts a boy who is dangerously sick with scarlet fever. When the boy begins to recover, the doctor orders that family burn the child's toys to kill the germs. The boy's favorite velveteen rabbit is sent to the pyre, but the boy's love transforms the toy into a living bunny. Today, a less remembered element of the story is what happens to the boy as he convalesces: the doctor sends the child to the beach to restore his health.[4]

Around the turn of the twentieth century, painters joined authors in depicting children at the beach, and among those artists were Americans George

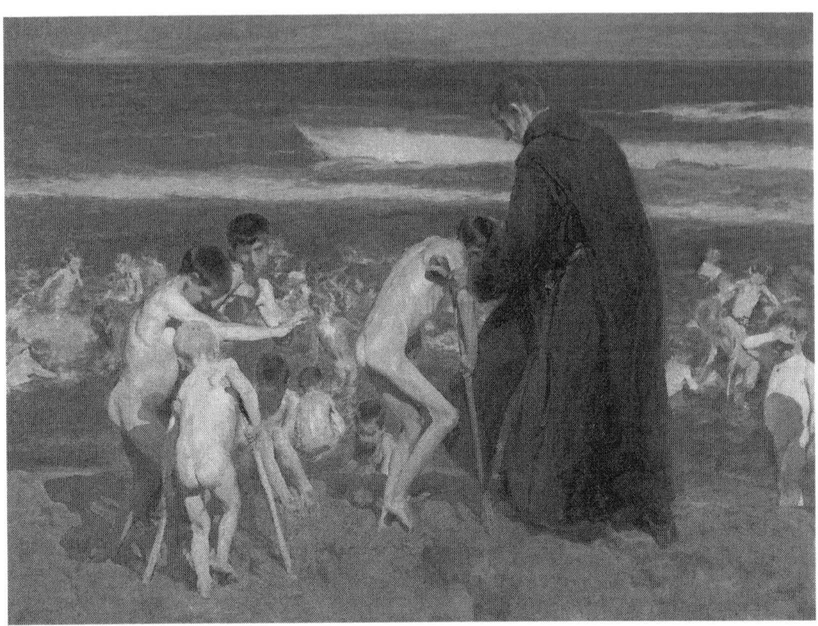

FIGURE 11. Joaquín Sorolla, *Sad Inheritance*, 1899. This painting shows a priest overseeing the "marine medication" of young patients with a range of health conditions. Public domain.

Bellows and Edward Henry Potthast, as well as Spanish painter Joaquín Sorolla. Sorolla's 1899 painting *Sad Inheritance* captures one such scene. The large canvas invites viewers to witness a large group of boys taking advantage of the seaside's therapeutic nature. Their naked bodies bear the marks of disease. One frail child crumples over a crutch, relying on a priest's assistance to navigate the sand. The boy's skin stretches against his bones, and his legs bend awkwardly as he struggles toward the ocean. Another child hobbles on his crutches, while an older boy appears to assist. Other, apparently healthier, children play in the waves beyond. Their nakedness not only demonstrates an unremarkable way of bathing for the time but also suggests an embrace of exposure as being therapeutic.[5]

The art community celebrated the painting. Sorolla won multiple awards, including the grand prize at the Exposition Universelle in Paris in 1900.[6]

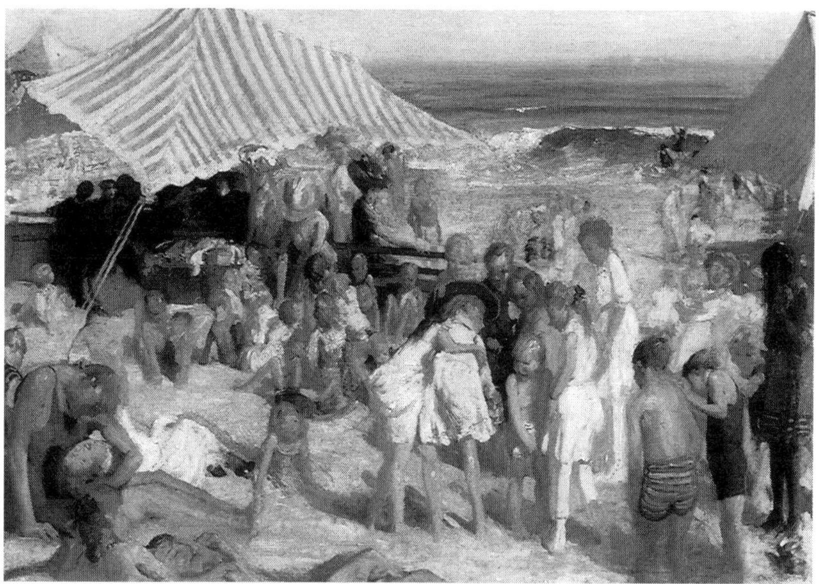

FIGURE 12. George Bellows, *Beach at Coney Island,* 1908. This painting features a bustling beach scene in which children figure prominently. Note the contrast with Bellows's depiction of children in his *Forty-Two Kids* (fig. 13), painted the previous year. Universal Images Group North America LLC/Alamy Stock Photo.

Sorolla reported that he had witnessed the scene while on the beach in Valencia. He had been sketching local fishermen when he noticed the group of naked children overseen by a single priest. Curious, he inquired what was happening and learned the children were patients at the Hospital of San Juan de Dios, an institution dedicated to caring for both destitute patients and those with disabilities.[7]

George Bellows was also captivated by children. Contemporaries knew Bellows for his depictions of gritty realities of everyday, working-class urban life. In 1908, he shifted his viewers' gazes from the city to the shore when he painted *Beach at Coney Island.* His depiction caused a stir. One critic characterized it as a "distinctly vulgar scene," perhaps the result of the adult couple who lounge in an amorous embrace in the lower left of the canvas.[8] Other adults dot the landscape, but children dominate. Some gather in groups, one seems intrigued

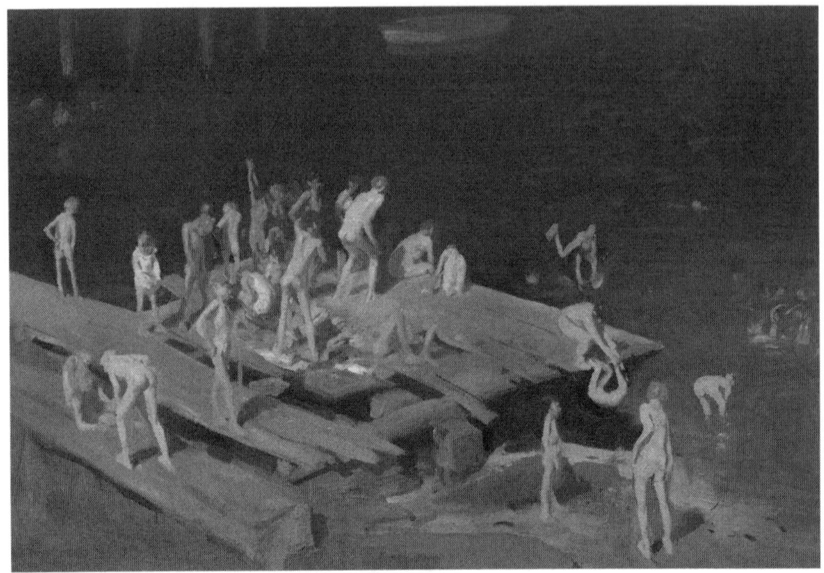

FIGURE 13. George Bellows, *Forty-Two Kids*, 1907. This dark painting is a stark contrast to the bright depiction of Coney Island, and it aligns with cultural associations of the city as unhealthy. SJ Art/Alamy Stock Photo.

by the viewer, others lie in the sand, and still more play in the waves. A baby clings to a woman's neck, while another bunch of children cluster beneath a striped tent as a woman in a long white dress and a wide-brimmed hat tends to them. Lovers aside, the beach is clearly a place for children.

Health interventions appear more subtly in Bellows's painting than in Sorolla's. Nevertheless, the American painter, like his Spanish counterpart, depicts a bright day, the beach lit by the sun, which the viewer cannot see. The scene suggests that the children enjoy the healthful effects of the seashore. In contrast, Bellows's 1907 oil painting, titled *Forty-Two Kids*, presents an image of young bathers in low light. A group of partially clad boys dive, lounge, chat, and swim on a dilapidated pier in the East River in New York City. The children may play, but the murky water and dark atmosphere suggest that health cannot, and will not, be found by these city kids.

Paintings and stories can tell us what adults believed about children's place at the seashore and offer hints about how children might have experienced the beach. Because children seldom leave written records, we must interpret sources produced by adults. Children of course have important stories to tell and perspectives all their own, but adults do not often preserve them. Parents discard the flotsam of childhood as babies become toddlers and then children, teenagers, and adults. What families keep, librarians and archivists catalog, and historians analyze reflects what society has recorded as relevant.[9] It is why we know so much about the Founding Fathers, luminary figures, and the "firsts" in their fields. It is also why we know far less about the women, mothers, and children who helped create and maintain the structures of society, while cultivating cultures of their own.

Like archaeologists, we can unearth fragments of information and piece together stories.[10] If we allow ourselves to imagine the seashore through the eyes of a child, we can understand how the beach could have been a space of fun and merriment, even for those debilitated by city life. To access what children may have experienced, we can examine the buildings, infrastructures, and activities created for them.[11] Doing so also gives us insight into prevailing cultural ideologies and the ways in which America's children shaped the seashore.[12]

Consider a child who came from the stoop of a bar, like Mamie Donoghy from chapter 1 or one of the forty-two kids from Bellows's painting. The seashore would have provided a striking contrast to their everyday lives. At the beach children would not have to dangle their feet from rotting wood that extended over filthy water, beneath polluted skies, to go swimming. At the shore they experienced abundant sun, seawater, and sand. Police did not arrest boys for playing on the beachfront of seashore hospitals as they did when children frolicked on the city streets. At the seashore adults encouraged children to run races and play games. Urban children who cared for younger siblings, assisted with chores, or worked for wages likely felt the joy and freedom of the beach even more acutely than their well-off counterparts.

Tens of thousands of children across the northeastern seaboard shared similar experiences after admission to pediatric seashore hospitals. As noted in the previous chapter, mothers brought children who were not acutely ill but persistently weak and thin. Other children arrived without maternal oversight.

For this class of patients, the seashore may have felt more like a summer camp than a hospitalization.[13] They maintained a schedule of healthful activities. For them, balneotherapy meant swimming in the ocean, and while playing outside with other children they would be getting their sea-air baths. When traveling from the city to the shore, they carried with them the idea that a trip to a beach was healthy because it was fun.

More concretely, images and texts show how adults constructed the notion of the beach as therapeutic for children because it provided opportunities for recreation, amusement, and play in healthy environments. Nevertheless, we must remain skeptical of adults' claims about the purity of children's pleasure. I do not argue that the managers of seashore hospitals spun tall tales, but they did use advertisements and annual reports to raise funds for their institutions. They promoted patients' happiness because it reflected popular and medical conceptions of the seashore's health-giving properties and its ability to rebuild bodies through familiar tourist practices.

Institutions' stories often accurately captured daily life for short-term summertime patients. Yet for children with chronic conditions, a stay at a hospital involved more time spent undergoing conventional therapeutic procedures than playing in the sand. Patients spent weeks and months strapped to backboards or confined in casts. They endured surgeries and separation from their families. Medical staff tried to provide amusement and education to children undergoing treatment. But given the duration and nature of the required treatments, lessons and fun activities represented a small portion of the children's hospitalization experience.

By the mid-twentieth century, children with chronic conditions who stayed at seaside hospitals had more in common with young patients undergoing urban hospitalization than with children experiencing the merriments of marine medication. Most health care occurred within the hospital walls, not outside on the beach. Relatively healthy children still went to institutions, including the Children's Seashore House, during the summer and spent much of their days outdoors. For these youth, play hid the fact that a day on the beach was both medicinal and preventive care. Later, as adults, they carried with them the idea that the seashore was a place where children could play and amusements were healing.

Pleasure and Play, Measured in Pounds

As more American families moved into cities, many parents no longer saw their children as important contributors to the family's economic well-being. As sociologists and historians have argued, the turn of the twentieth century was a moment when upper- and middle-class Americans began to embrace their children as sentimentally precious and priceless.[14] Around the same time, psychologists and physicians began to study children, and they promoted childhood as a separate developmental life stage. They advanced ideas that children had unique needs that changed as they grew.

As we learned in chapter 1, professionals and parents advocated that time spent outside in natural settings improved children's health. They also agreed that cities lacked these necessary environments. Adults saw cities as artificial, technological, and therefore unnatural, spaces. Psychologists, pediatricians, and child welfare advocates argued that children suffered as a result of the dislocation from natural settings.[15]

Ideas about childhood and the seashore progressed in tandem. Around the same time that Dr. Jonathan Pitney arrived on Absecon Island, psychologists, physicians, and politicians looked at children and determined youth needed special attention to grow and attain their potential.[16] They constructed the seashore as a place where urban children could develop into healthy, productive adults.

Doctors argued that healthy environments combated a generalized mental illness they associated with urban living. According to prominent physicians, the excitement and stimulation of city life negatively affected children's developing brains. L. Emmett Holt, one of the country's first pediatricians and a founder of the American Pediatric Society, argued that children's brains were uniquely sensitive to external stimuli.[17] Holt advocated for children to be protected against "not only tea, coffee, and alcohol, but undue and unnatural excitement." He wrote that "normal development can take place only in the midst of quiet and peaceful surroundings. The conditions of modern life, especially in cities, are such that these laws are almost invariably violated, and the consequences of this are seen in the marked and steady increase in nervous diseases among children of all classes."[18] Holt's claims aligned with more general concerns about the depleting effects of the city; around the same time, doctors defined neurasthenia as a disease that adults developed as a result of the enervating forces of city life.

Holt advocated for removing children from the environment that made them agitated, writing, "Altogether the most satisfactory way of bringing up such a child is in the country away from the excitement and distractions of city life."[19] Of course few families could permanently relocate, but as we have seen, many took advantage of nonurban institutions like seashore hospitals, health homes, or expansive parks, such as that provided by the Sanitarium Association of Philadelphia.

One Philadelphia family's story is instructive for understanding how children moved between their urban homes and institutions located in healthier environments. In 1921, a social worker from the Hospital of the University of Pennsylvania made her way to a bicycle shop in Philadelphia to follow up on a young patient named Abraham. She knew he was a tough case. Abraham had not fully recovered before leaving the hospital, and the social worker had previously flagged Abraham for his bad attitude and foul language. Arriving at the shop, the social worker discovered that the family lived in "very poor dark rooms" and had problems that extended beyond Abraham's ill health. Abraham's father had lost his job at Baldwin's, a Philadelphia-based locomotive manufacturer. The family had limited funds as a result of purchasing stock for the bicycle shop. The social worker discovered that Abraham was still unhealthy. A physician had recommended that the boy receive convalescent care that included fresh air and good food.[20]

Abraham would have to leave his home in the city to fill the doctor's prescription. The social worker reached out to the Children's Seashore House in Atlantic City and requested admission and financial assistance. The physicians there granted her request, and Abraham left for the hospital by the sea. Abraham had returned home by March the following year. The social worker made her way back to the bicycle shop to check on the child. She felt pleased, and perhaps even surprised, at Abraham's transformation, noting she had "never seen a child so improved, both physically and mentally, by an outing. He looked and acted like a different boy, and was in such good spirits." She worried that his return to the city would jeopardize his health, however, lamenting, "The home is a very poor one, and the mother, tho devoted, seems to have very little control of him." She wondered, in her notes, about the benefits of sending Abraham to the country for further benefit.[21]

Transformations like Abraham's were common, according to Dr. William Bennett. As Bennett neared his fortieth year at the Children's Seashore House, he reflected on his institution's work. He found it difficult to capture patients' experience: "no figures can give an idea of the many wondrous changes wrought from feebleness to health or tell of the days of happiness and sufficiency given to hundreds into whose lives at home comes but little mental sunshine, and for whose growing bodies there is very often too little good nutritious food."[22] Physicians celebrated the physical and emotional transformations that resulted from time spent in the salubrious environment at the seashore.

Pediatric patients seemed to embrace the opportunities presented by seashore hospitals. While some parents may have cajoled their children into going to the institutions, the sheer number of visitors supports the conclusion that children reported positive experiences during their hospital stays. Adults who had spent time at the Children's Seashore House in their youth sometimes sent their own children. In 1910, Bennett described multigenerational admissions as one of the institution's successes: "To more than forty thousand poor children of Philadelphia the Children's House has proved a Paradise. They have loved it. Many of them have come again and again, and now some of its early guests are sending their children to the place where they were happy and grew strong."[23] Looking back as adults, former patients may have remembered their time fondly and wanted to share that experience with their own children.

While it can be tempting to dismiss Bennett's claims as hyperbole meant to inspire donations, other sources offer confirming evidence. Even those urban children who had never visited the beach longed to go, suggesting they had positive associations with the shore. As discussed in chapter 4, the children in the 1881 illustration captioned "Summer Resorts of the Poor," longed to go to the beach.

Such stories suggest that working-class children knew the beach as a place of play where they could seek relief from the difficulties of urban life. While most working-class children could not experience summer-long sojourns to the sea like some upper-class children, those who went to seashore hospitals learned that the beach was a place they belonged. They absorbed the knowledge that laughter and hurrahs, like swimming in the ocean, eating good food, and bathing in the fresh air and sunlight, were beneficial.

Connecting Health and Play at the Shore

Children from wealthier families might enjoy a vacation at the beach, such as the fictional characters in the Bobbsey Twins and Honey Bunch series of books. American impressionist painter Edward Henry Potthast portrayed many moments of seemingly well-to-do children playing and enjoying time wading in the ocean under bright sunshine.

Working-class children also went to the beach. Families might have been able to afford day trips, but children traveling alone could access more beach time at seaside hospitals. Like mothers who stayed at cottages on hospital grounds, working-class children's robust presence at hospitals reinforced associations of the beach as a therapeutic destination, because it gave them a safe place to play.

Many summertime patients arrived at the Children's Seashore House without an acute illness but were rather run-down or noted as having debility. When they arrived at the beach, they discovered they would enjoy ample time to play outside, and they learned that amusements characterized their time at the seashore. In July 1901, nine-year-old Victoria and her thirteen-year-old sister Maizie went to the Children's Seashore House.[24] Neither child was sick per se, but they had traveled from their home in Philadelphia to Atlantic City anyway. The same week Victoria and Maizie arrived, at least five other groups of sisters also made the journey to the hospital.[25] Some of those girls were noted as being "delicate," two had headaches, and one, Rosie, had bronchitis. None was seriously ill.[26]

Maizie and Victoria likely traveled by train and then boarded an ambulance that carried them down the beach to the new hospital building. The girls would have entered the main entrance, where a nurse collected their admissions cards. Victoria's card recorded that she had debility and was free of contagious diseases. Since the sisters were there without their mother, they stayed in a large ward in the main building with other girls of their age.

Victoria and Maizie would have followed a routine during their ten days at the hospital. They woke early and ate breakfast in a large dining hall with other patients. Meals included generous portions of milk, eggs, oatmeal, fruit, and vegetables.[27] After breakfast, the head nurse read prayers, and then the children returned to their ward, where they waited for the doctor to examine them.

After the physician's visit, the children played at the beach until lunch, which they ate at 10:00 a.m. Everyone was back outside by 11:00 a.m. Nurses gathered children in groups and sent them for a swim. Victoria and Maizie would have held the hands of the children next to them as they waded into the waves until the nurse called them to shore. After their sea-bath, Victoria, Maizie, and the other children played outside, breaking for supper at 12:30 and dinner at 5:30 p.m.[28] One report indicated a dinner menu of roast beef and potatoes.[29] At bedtime, they returned to the wards, where the open windows allowed sea breezes to blow over the sleeping children all night.

Victoria and Maizie spent more than a week at the seashore. They, like the other groups of sisters, benefited from their stay. All of the girls were "well" when they left the hospital. Even Rosie, the girl who had arrived with bronchitis, left the hospital in good health.[30]

We may not know exactly how Victoria or Maizie felt before, during, or after their stay at the Children's Seashore House. It is possible that for each girl, being with her sister brought them a sense of comfort; children at other institutions reported as much.[31] Meeting other groups of siblings who also arrived without parents and were not critically ill may have framed the experience less as a hospitalization and more like a summer camp. The routines, common dining, play time, and even prayers mirrored daily life at other camps, although at the time there were few such institutions for girls.[32] Regardless, the hours children enjoyed playing on the sandy beachfront of the hospital would stand in stark contrast to daily life in the city.

Tens of thousands of urban children experienced the beach through a hospital, which linked play, health care, and the seashore. In 1913, Dr. Bennett explained that happiness was of equal importance in nature-based therapies and nutritional needs: "For all of our children our aim is to provide all the sunshine and fresh air obtainable; all the *appetizing* nutritious food that can be digested, and all the happiness that can be devised. Toys, laughter, singing and hurrahs are part of the treatment, a Psychotherapy which greatly aids our Thalasso-therapy."[33] Happiness, in this physician's estimate, provided children with the most comprehensive care possible. In addition to daily play on the beach, pediatric patients went to the amusements on the piers, including shows, movies, and mazes, carnival rides. Once a week, the patients enjoyed front-row seats at "the exhibit of the trained birds and lions," on Young's Pier. They also rode the trolley cars and ate candy from the vendors on the piers.[34] Donors gave money for chicken dinners and ice cream parties, while musicians, jazz bands, and circuses performed at the hospital.[35]

It is unclear if children would have understood their time at seaside hospitals as being medicinal or therapeutic. Doctors may have heralded the benefits of "thalasso-therapy," but children may have just seen it as swimming. Of course they would be aware they were at a hospital and that nurses and physicians monitored their well-being. But it seems likely that their primary experience was that the beach was a place to play with other children, outdoors in the sand and surf. Feeling better, particularly for those who were not critically or chronically ill, may have been a secondary consideration.

When the Children's Seashore House opened a summer camp for boys in 1897, it reinforced the connections between recreation and the beach. Summer camps had risen in popularity around this time. Initially only children from wealthy families could access camps in the nineteenth century. The Young Men's Christian Association (YMCA) established camps for middle-class boys in the 1890s, thereby extending access to more youth. By 1905, YMCAS were operating 178 camps in the United States. Organizers, benefactors, and counselors worked to instill campers with a sense of rugged masculinity, a reflection of professionals' and politicians' fretting that modern city life and "brain-work" produced weak, even feminine, men.[36]

Psychologists such as G. Stanley Hall promoted interventions that exposed boys to rough-and-tumble experiences. Encouraging boys to act out the role of "savages," so the thinking went, would allow them to develop into stronger men who could withstand the depleting forces of civilized adult life.[37] Camps operated on the assumption that time outside the city, in nature, would strengthen children in body and spirit. Proponents of summer camps argued that physical activity in the fresh air, as well as camaraderie forged around dining tables and campfires, restored the vitality and spirit drained by urban life.

This focus on restoring health for urban youth aligned with the mission of the Children's Seashore House. Opening a camp also solved a long-standing issue for the hospital: it had previously banned older boys, fearing they would be a disruptive and negative influence on the other patients.

Boys came to the first season of the Children's Seashore House summer camp in 1897. Most of the children were "in fair health who merely needed a little change"; like many of the children admitted to mothers' cottages, they were not suffering from disease.[38] When boys reached the camp, they saw a permanent wooden structure that served as the camp kitchen, complete with plumbing and water from Atlantic City. Nearby, tents stood on platforms, ensuring that campers would stay dry during storms. One large tent operated as the dining room, while another held twenty cots for sleeping.[39]

Campers led busy lives. They bathed in the ocean, reportedly enjoying "this sport to the full." Every day boys would pull *Jennie*, the rowboat, into the breakers. Hopping into the boat, they rowed the quarter of a mile to the main hospital building, where they gathered provisions for the day before returning to their campsite. Boys could also take the rowboat into the water to fish and crab. Some campers even had an opportunity to ride aboard a sloop. The boys filled two such boats and egged on the "experienced sea captains," requesting that they turn the afternoon into a "prolonged yacht race." The captains obliged, to the boys' delight.[40]

Outings and sporting events punctuated campers' experiences and instilled in them the idea that the beach was a place for recreation. Boys played baseball with nearby teams and organized a series of games against the resident doctors of the Children's Seashore House. The campers held track meets complete with relay teams. The "captain" who oversaw the camp even allowed the boys to explore Atlantic City and the boardwalk, as long as the campers returned in time for supper. As the day wound down, campers gathered around the campfire, where "the time passed with stories and songs." A bit before 9:00 p.m., the boys meandered from the fire pit to their tents. Tired from their day outside in the seawater, sea breezes, and sunshine, everyone was "mighty glad to turn in."[41]

The camp quickly gained popularity. In 1898, a donor gave money for a second tent, and that year eighty-six boys spent a few weeks camping at the seashore. Physicians and donors were impressed by the boys' health improvements. Some campers gained quite a bit of weight during their stays. On average each child gained three to four pounds, and one boy left camp eight pounds heavier than when he arrived. The boys who were the weakest at admission might make the biggest recoveries. As the doctor at the main hospital recorded, "The great improvement in the condition of one or two real invalids showed that it [the camp] possessed possibilities for usefulness beyond what we expected."[42]

When children camped at the Children's Seashore House, the experience presumably bore little resemblance to hospitalization. Rather, their experiences had more in common with those of middle- and upper-class children who attended other camps. Since most children were not sick, their time at the hospital camp promoted a sense that the beach was a place to have fun, be active, and enjoy the camaraderie of other boys. The summer camp conveyed the message to working-class children that they benefited from staying at the seashore and playing in the sand and water. When those patients returned home, they carried the knowledge that the beach was a space where children belonged.

Smiling Joe

Most of the patients at the Children's Seashore House were similar to the boys at the camp or the girls like Victoria and Maizie: urban children who weren't acutely or chronically sick but could benefit and grow stronger at the health-giving seashore. However, American seashore hospitals also cared for pediatric patients with serious, chronic medical conditions. Many of these patients suffered from tuberculosis that had attacked their joints and spines, causing them to double over. Others arrived with bones weakened from rickets, their legs bowing under the weight of their torsos. Infantile paralysis (polio) had paralyzed other patients.

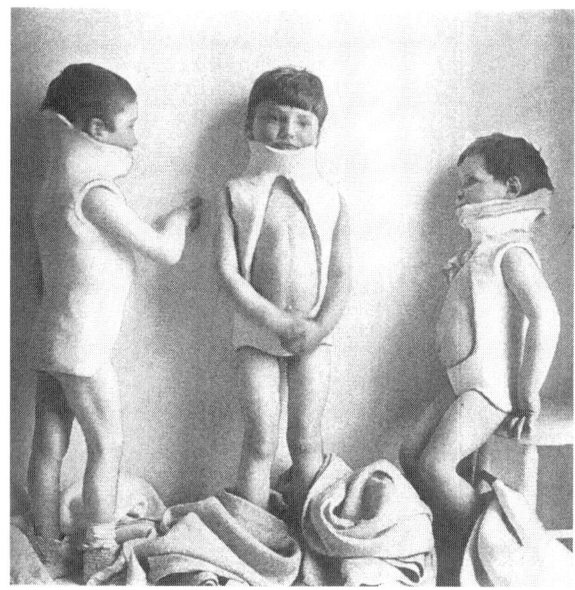

FIGURE 14. Pediatric patients at Sea Breeze Hospital in plaster casts with windows to allow for sun exposure. In Guy Hinsdale, *Atmospheric Air in Relation to Tuberculosis* (Washington, DC: Smithsonian Institution, 1914), plate 16.

Unsurprisingly, these children's experiences differed from the children who came for a short respite or a week at camp. Patients with chronic conditions stayed for months or even years. Family may have visited, but they certainly could not remain for the duration of a patient's stay. For children with orthopedic conditions, physicians supplemented marine medication with devices like Bradford frames, which required children to be strapped to an arched board throughout the day. Other patients sported casts that extended from their chins to their waists. Pleasure and play did not define these patients' experiences.

Yet hospital boosters championed the idea that these patients experienced happiness and joy. They shared tales of children who were rescued from death's bony grip and who appreciated the opportunity to heal while enjoying special parties, taking treks along the boardwalk, playing games, and spending time with visiting dignitaries. Patients were happy, reports claimed, because they were healing at the seashore.

Administrators at the Sea Breeze hospital in Coney Island painted this rosy picture with success. The hospital had first opened in 1903 as a tent colony. A

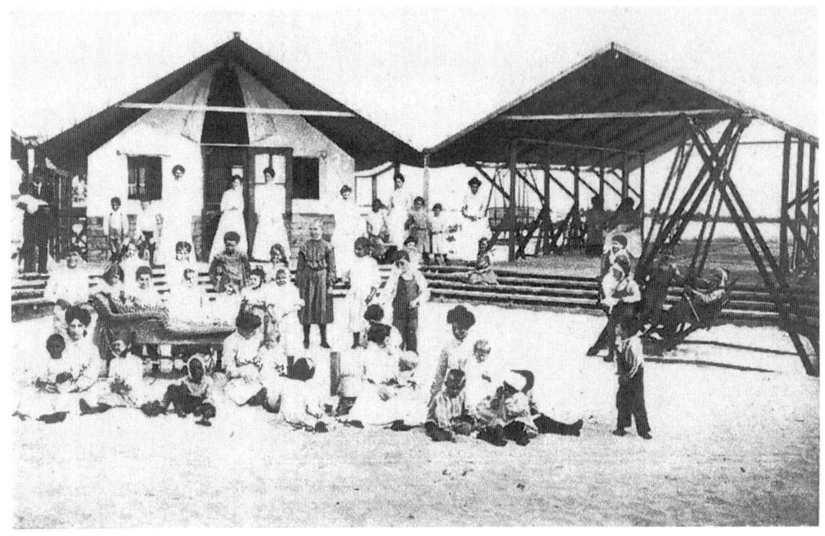

FIGURE 15. Early photograph of Sea Breeze as a tent hospital. Note the children from different races, with a range of physical abilities, and the women overseeing children. In Guy Hinsdale, *Atmospheric Air in Relation to Tuberculosis* (Washington, DC: Smithsonian Institution, 1914), plate 10.

board member of the Association for Improving the Condition of the Poor recommended establishing a permanent institution after traveling to Europe, where he visited a pediatric seashore hospital and was impressed by its results. By 1904, the association had raised money and built a permanent institution that cared for New York City's tubercular children. Tourists lined the fences of Sea Breeze to watch patients play in the sun and sand.[43]

Patient demand quickly outstripped the first hospital's capacity. Hospital administrators enlisted the help of one of their patients with nonpulmonary tuberculosis, "Smiling Joe," to raise funds for a larger building. As mentioned in chapter 2, Smiling Joe captured public attention and headlines in the early twentieth century when he became one of the hospital's first year-round patients. The public learned that the seashore coupled happiness and healing for the young child. A news article in *World Events* reported that Joe's "back was twisted by bone tuberculosis," while another explained, "When Joe came he had tubercular glands in his back and could scarcely crawl. He was in danger of being bent almost double."[44] Physicians strapped Joe to an arched board to straighten his spine. He remained on the board for one year. Once Joe's spine had recovered, doctors fitted a "tight plaster cast" that covered his torso, with openings at the front and back designed to allow sunlight to penetrate his skin and kill subcutaneous bacteria. Joe wore the cast for three years. During this time, the public read stories about Joe "playing about the beach as best he could in his tight-fitting jacket in the daytime, and sleeping in a dormitory with large windows thrown wide open during the summer and winter."[45]

Ad campaigns highlighted Joe's sunny disposition, but the images belied a much more arduous existence. Joe's treatment took four years. During this time he was bound to or enclosed in orthopedic devices. At best it would seem

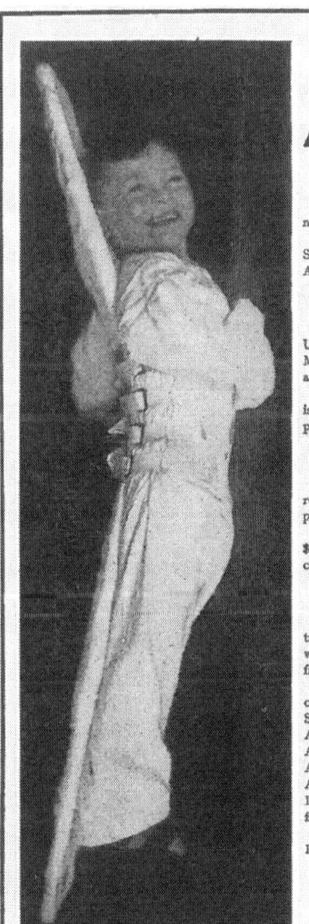

A Cheerful View
of
A Serious Situation

Situation I.

Crippled by bone tuberculosis, strapped to a board night and day.

Joe smiles because he is being wonderfully cured at Sea Breeze, by the outdoor salt air treatment, the first American temporary hospital for such cases.

Situation II.

4,500 such children in New York, 60,000 in the United States, *only 44* at Sea Breeze. Five-year-old Max speaks for all, "I don't want to get dead and be an angel, I want to play first."

Joe smiles again because the large permanent hospital is already planned, to save many more from a life of pain and uselessness.

Situation III.

Of the $250,000 needed for this hospital $35,000 remains to be raised at once, or the sums already pledged *may be lost*.

Joe's smile is a hurry call to you for a part of this $35,000. The money can't wait, Joe can't wait, the crippled children tortured in the tenements can't wait.

Situation IV.

Sea Breeze is also the place where the Association is trying to provide Fresh Air for 20,000 others, many of whom are sick or at the breaking point, with no escape from dark, foul tenements and stifling streets.

Buy happiness for them, with strength and new courage, by sending to Sea Breeze for a week

Some overworked mother with four children,	$10.00
A teething baby and "little mother" of ten,	5.00
An underfed shop girl earning $3.00 per week,	2.50
An aged woman fighting for self-support,	2.50
A day party of 400, for one glorious day,	100 00

Leave happiness behind, it will catch up. Send 2 cents for Happiness Calendar.

Hurry check or pledge to R. S. Minturn, Treasurer, Room 203, No. 105 East 22d Street, New York City.

New York Association for Improving the Condition of the Poor

R. Fulton Cutting, Pres.

1843-1906

FIGURE 16. A published appeal for donations included this image of the child known as "Smiling Joe," a tuberculosis patient strapped to a backboard. Author's collection.

dull and uncomfortable, and at worst excruciating and painful. Joe endured physical hardships and separation from his family. Yet reporters promoted images of healing, physical rehabilitation, and encouraging smiles, thereby deepening cultural associations of the seashore's capacity to heal and inspire happiness even among the sickest patients.

Smiling Joe became a champion of Sea Breeze and a poster boy for marine medication more broadly. A newspaper article bolstered these associations. In 1905, the *New York World* reported that Theodore Roosevelt walked through the hospital and came to Joe's bed. One of the physicians introduced Roosevelt to the boy, saying "'This is little Joe Marion. . . . He is suffering from tuberculosis of the spine, but we expect to cure him.' 'Poor little fellow,' said the President, and his eyes welled up with tears." True to form, Joe "broke into a smile." The doctor explained, "'He always smiles. . . . That's why we call him 'Smiling Joe.'"[46] Before leaving that day, Roosevelt stood outside and looked at the ocean. Inspired by the patients and hospital's seaside location he exclaimed, "'Ha . . . they can't help getting well here.'"[47]

Recognizing Joe's ability to inspire, the Association for Improving the Condition of the Poor circulated a photograph of Joe and his famous grin.[48] In the picture, Joe is wrapped tightly in white cloth from his neck down to his toes. His arms, encased in fabric, are crossed upon his chest. A separate cloth device encircles Joe's stomach and chest, strapping him to the board. Joe's body arches backward, but he beams at the camera. The bright and broad smile on his cherubic face defies his confinement. His round, ruddy cheeks reassured viewers that the seashore cured.

In June 1906, Sea Breeze administrators reinforced the seashore as a restorative site when they published a full-page advertisement entitled "A Cheerful View of a Serious Situation" in the *New York Observer*. A photograph of "Smiling Joe" appears on the left side of the ad, and the Association for Improving the Condition of the Poor reassured the public that Joe was smiling because the salt air treatment was curing him.[49] But the text of the ad alerts readers that there were forty-five hundred children in New York City and sixty thousand children in the United States who needed the same care as Joe.[50] Yet Sea Breeze could admit "*only 44*" given the hospital's space limitations.[51] The foundation pleaded with donors for the final $35,000 they needed to build a larger hospital and serve more children. Trying to encourage donations, they explained that "the money can't wait, Joe can't wait, the crippled children tortured in the tenements can't wait." Offering a supporting voice, a five-year-old boy named Max implored, "I don't want to get dead and be an angel, I want to play first."[52]

These words highlighted patients' awareness of their health conditions and prognoses. Children knew they were sick and could die. Such insights, and children's articulate expressions of their conditions, inspired a who's who of New Yorkers to donate. The *New York Times* reported that John D. Rockefeller offered to give $125,000 toward a new hospital but only if an equivalent amount could be raised by the end of the year.[53] Sea Breeze achieved this objective in the nick of time: on December 31, 1905, George H. F. Schrader gave the remaining $19,850 to reach the goal. In addition to Rockefeller and Schrader, other prominent members of society donated to Sea Breeze, including Andrew Carnegie, Murry Guggenheim, and Joseph Pulitzer.[54] Hundreds of ordinary citizens and children joined these social elites, donating what they could.

Newspaper articles and flyers continued to celebrate Joe's recovery and spread the word that the seashore could cure severely ill patients. They reported that after four years Joe's spine had straightened and he was able to "walk and run about like other children."[55] Marine medication, with an assist by orthopedic devices, cured Joe.

In 1909, the *New York Times* feted Joe's $250,000 smile and his transformation into a robust and healthy child. The article detailed a host of other children whose recoveries were "quite as remarkable" as Joe's, including

> Agnes and her chum, Madeline, who may be seen jumping rope up and down the beach at Sea Breeze. Both had tuberculosis of the spine, and when Agnes was brought there, she was declared "marked for certain death" by the dispensary from which she came, but Agnes is almost well now, after a course of sea air and good food.
>
> Jacob, the champion leap-frog player of Sea Breeze, is another notable recovery. His trouble was in his right leg, and it was supposed that only amputation could save him. The boy was suffering so intensely that he

had to be taken to Coney Island in an automobile specially padded and cushioned. Jacob's right foot isn't entirely well yet, but he is so strong that, in spite of it, he indulges in all kinds of activities, leap-frog being his specialty.

> Margaret is a little black-haired Irish girl whose ankle was said to demand immediate amputation. She was sent down to be strengthened for the operation, but the course of eggs, milk, and salt water bathing worked wonders. She has been sent home cured, but that doesn't prevent her slipping down to Sea Breeze on every possible occasion to play with the swings. Glorying in her strength, Margaret scorns to sit down and swing quietly. She stands up, grasping the ropes and "pumps" for the little girls who are still wearing their plaster casts.[56]

Play figured prominently in children's stories of recovery. Agnes and Madeline jumped rope together, while Jacob loved playing leapfrog. Margaret's story conveys the fondness that children had for the institution and the opportunities for fun it presented. Even after children went home, they returned to swing with the patients who remained.

When Joe had recovered and prepared to leave the hospital, newspapers reported that he "took all the children who were able" to the circus, including Jacob, Agnes, and Madeline, noted above, as well as twelve other patients. They arrived at the big tent in Brooklyn for the Ringling Brothers' performance. The children took delight in the "ladies who floated in the air" and the clown-policeman who "made a great many arrests for the especial benefit of Joe's party." The pinnacle of the show came "when one clown stole another clown's balloons and was suddenly hoisted in the air, presumably by the balloons, only to fall into the policeman's hands later when the balloons broke away, and the clown came to the ground."[57] At the end of the evening, Joe returned to Sea Breeze with his comrades for his final night. When Joe left the next day, he "rode away on horseback in front of one of the mounted police at Coney Island to great applause."[58]

The public remained intrigued by Joe's story. They learned that he returned to his home in New York City's East Side after physicians discharged him from Sea Breeze. Three years later, the *Washington Post* reported that "Smiling

Joe is a sturdy little youth of 10 years, living with his parents," and attending his local school. His teacher gushed, "There isn't a happier boy in the school than Joe Marion. Except when he is studying hard he is always laughing."[59]

The popular interest in Joe's story fits within the cultural investment in children's health and new medical interventions, as previously discussed. However, unlike incubator shows that displayed technological marvels, the stories of children at seashore hospitals reinforced medical and vernacular knowledge that the seashore healed not only by dosing nature but also by encouraging play and happiness. When newspapers highlighted stories of presidential visits and circus trips, leapfrog and swings, they solidified cultural associations of the beach as a place where play was restorative.

Smiling Joe likely represented more of an amalgam of adults' ideas and promotional campaigns rather than a patient whom the public truly knew. Historians and scholars of childhood have argued that the stories adults tell about children often reveal more about prevailing cultural values than they do about children's lived experiences and beliefs.[60] Joe represented what people wanted to believe: that the seashore healed by making people happy. His smile testified to this fact. Yet the tales newspapers told obscured the difficulties of prolonged institutionalization and instead pulled the public's attention to the power of the seashore to heal the sickest urban children.

No Day at the Beach

There are few firsthand written accounts from children about their time at seashore hospitals. One that still exists is a diary kept by Howard Gershenfeld, who spent eight months as a pediatric patient at the Children's Seashore House beginning in 1939 and extending into 1940. His written record of his experience provides a more nuanced look into children's lives during long-term stays. His words capture the trials and tears that accompanied the circuses and celebrations; they also suggest that by the mid-twentieth century the beach had receded from the center of medical practice, replaced by procedures and drugs administered indoors.

The diary begins on January 1, 1940. Taking out his new "Five Year Diary," Howard looked at the four short lines he had to record his thoughts. Picking up his pencil, he jotted, "We had a chicken dinner and later the xmas tree was taken down. I heard the Rose Bowl Game."[61] The USC Trojans beat the Tennessee Volunteers, 14–0.[62]

Similar scenes may have played out in houses across America, but Howard had spent his New Year's Day at the Children's Seashore House in Atlantic City. He had been at the hospital since July, when he had been transferred from Jefferson Hospital in Philadelphia. Howard had rheumatic endocarditis, a condition that weakens the heart valves. He first received care in the city and then moved to the Children's Seashore House during the summer to further recover.

Howard recorded his impressions in his diary until he left the Children's Seashore House on March 9, 1940. Medical procedures earn less mention than one might expect; Howard tended to note special events or treats. Given what adults wrote about children's experiences at seashore hospitals in the early twentieth century, this pattern in Howard's diary could suggest that his account affirms adults' claims about play and entertainment. However, a close reading of Howard's diary reveals that he likely centered these events because they were out of the ordinary.

The diary hints at discontent and unhappiness, implied by what and how he recorded each day's events. One day Howard wrote that a Dr. Rise performed a procedure on a fellow patient's "leg and it bled a lot."[63] Howard seemed uncomfortable when Rise conducted a procedure on Eugene, another boy in the hospital. On February 3 Howard recorded, "For the second straight day Dr. Rise cut Eugene's leg. It happened at supper time and Eugene cried and screamed."[64] Howard's entries about Eugene, a regular recipient of invasive procedures, are some of the most difficult to read. Unlike the beaming smiles and sparkling sunshine of promotional texts, here the echoes of a child crying in agony make pediatric patients' discomfort visceral.

Yet advertisements and annual reports from earlier decades may not have totally misled readers. Howard also recorded moments of fun and heartfelt care. On January 15, Howard's shop teacher, Miss Roberts, returned from vacation.[65] Howard seemed happy that Roberts was back. Roberts looked out for Howard, entertaining him and his fellow patients. One night Howard wrote that she "played cards with John, Andy, and Me. They won."[66] On another occasion, Howard and Roberts played pinochle, and once Roberts hosted a party for the children in conjunction with Miss Knee, the ward nurse. Roberts also treated the boys to "strawberry ice cream pie and pretzel sticks."[67] Another time, she "brought John L. a candy hot dog." Howard reported that John let him eat half of it.[68]

The warmth Howard felt toward his shop teacher appears most vividly in his January 25 entry. On that night Roberts went to the ward expecting to play cards with some boys. It was a ruse. Instead of playing cards, Howard recorded that the patients had treated her to a surprise party to celebrate her birthday.[69]

Planning a surprise party suggests a meaningful relationship between patients and their providers. In this regard, Roberts was not the only person to earn the boys' respect. Howard and the other boys in the unit looked to Miss Knee as a source of care, stability, and authority. In some instances Knee acted like a parent. For instance, Howard recorded that Knee was frustrated by Irving, who ate more slowly than his peers. Knee resorted to bribery, promising Irving that if he could "eat all his meals in 30 minutes she'd get him a steak dinner."[70]

Knee also used rewards to shape children's behavior. Howard recorded that Knee promised the patients they would "see the World Series motion pictures next Tues. eve, if we were good."[71] Knee looked after the children in other ways as well. She had everyday conversations with the patients that ranged from impending nor'easters to upcoming visitors and appointments. She took care of their needs and tended to everyday illnesses. When Howard had a sore throat, Knee "painted it." When John L. became constipated, she gave him "milk of magnesia every night for a while."[72] And, as with parents, when she went away, the children misbehaved. On February 1, Knee took the afternoon off. In her absence Howard wrote that "the kids were bad."[73]

Although nurses fulfilled the everyday caregiving duties normally performed by mothers, patients felt their mothers' and fathers' absence. Howard was relatively fortunate in this regard. He saw either one or both of his parents almost every week. Over the course of the ten weeks that Howard remained in the hospital in 1940, he saw his father four times and his mother seven, not including the day he was discharged. In addition, Howard's uncles and siblings made the seventy-five-mile trip from Media, Pennsylvania, to visit him. They brought Howard gifts such as movie books, stamps, and letters.[74] Howard's family even took him out for a ride one Monday afternoon.[75] Other patients' parents also came to the hospital. Howard recorded that Irving's mother came and brought a chocolate bar.[76]

These visits, however, were fleeting, leaving nurses and staff to oversee children's care and well-being most of the time. When another patient, Edward John Hudak, reflected on the seven years that he spent at the Children's Seashore House, he recalled that "the dedicated staff adopted them all."[77] Edward initially went to the Atlantic City facility in the 1950s after he contracted polio. His doctor informed his parents that Edward's "chances for progress would be higher if my rehabilitation period was spent with people who were less emotionally involved and yet caring and professional."[78] Despite the recommended separation, Edward's parents drove sixty miles to see him most Sundays. Not all patients were so fortunate. Edward recalled that "some kids whose families lived at greater distances rarely had visitors." Staff helped fill the void. Still, Edward remembered his sadness at his parents' departures and how his homesickness never subsided.[79]

Edward spent much of the 1950s at the hospital, and, like Howard, he reflected on the special events and outings the hospital provided for him and his fellow patients. Edward recalled that "Christmas time was the best." In the weeks leading up to the holiday, various community and philanthropic groups would "show up each day with presents, ice cream, entertainment and Santa Claus. . . . And just when you thought you couldn't stomach another spoonful of ice cream or chorus of 'Jingle Bells,' the Ice Capades would hit town, and it was party time again." Nevertheless, Edward spent most of his days attending school and undergoing physical and occupational therapy.[80]

As an adult, Edward reminisced about his time at the Children's Seashore House, remembering both the pleasurable and the painful moments of his seven-year stay at the facility. Edward finally left the Atlantic City hospital in 1959, and he characterized the decision as much an emotional choice as a medical one. After spending seven years there he "was tired of the tear-filled Sunday afternoon partings. I wanted to go home, and the doctors agreed it was time." He left the "city I knew by the ocean" where he had spent so much of his childhood.[81]

Both Howard and Edward make clear that long-term patients appreciated moments of play and entertainment. Unsurprisingly, however, for children who lived in hospitals for months or years, tears and treatment defined their stays as much as parties and play. For these patients the seashore location was a backdrop to more modern medical practices.

Yet there were still vestiges of marine medication for patients who came for shorter stays in the warmer months. Despite the passage of decades, summer at the Children's Seashore House remained a time of amusement even into the 1950s. Edward recalled that "during the summer, Seashore House was a vacation resort for children with disabilities. All the dormitory-style rooms had French doors that opened to large verandas over-looking the beach and Boardwalk." As in previous decades, children paid little or nothing for their admission. Organizations, including the March of Dimes and the Ocean City Yacht Club, covered their costs. The yacht club went even further and provided patients with day-long trips on "big cabin cruisers," not unlike the sloop rides campers took fifty years earlier. In addition to sailing, the children enjoyed "picnics, theater trips, and all the attractions of Steel Pier."[82]

Entertainment continued to characterize the summer, maintaining the association between the seashore, health, and happiness. Yet for patients who remained for the winter months, like Howard, or for years, like Edward, the seashore was more a vista than a source of medicine. The beach no longer played a prominent role in these patients' health care regimens.

SEASHORE HOSPITALS PROVIDE INSIGHT into how thousands of working-class children learned that health might be regained through play in a natural environment like the beach. Institutions such as the Children's Seashore Hospital cultivated a camp- or vacation-like experience. Digging in the sand, swimming in the ocean, having holiday or birthday parties, playing baseball, and eating ice cream and fancy dinners all contributed to marine medication. As Dr. William Bennett wrote in 1914, "It is a doctrine of our

Institution that happiness is a most valuable factor in the restoration of the sick, and every effort is made to provide an atmosphere of it. The children talk, laugh, sing and shout without restraint."[83]

Many working-class urban children knew the seashore only through a hospital, where they spent a week playing with other children on the beach. They carried their experiences of the seashore as a space of pleasure and play back home to the city, where they spread knowledge throughout their families and communities. When relatively healthy children stayed at seaside hospitals, they learned that the beach was a place where children were free of many daily obligations and the dangers of street play. Their experiences of the shore had less to do with medical treatment than they did with being on the beach with friends and siblings. And yet their activities took place in a hospital environment. If hospitalized working-class patients primarily experienced the beach as entertaining, then children visiting the shore outside of institutional boundaries must have felt the connection between the seaside and leisure even more intensely.

As we learned from the young patients Howard and Edward, by the mid-twentieth century the seashore's landscape had become a backdrop to medical care for chronically ill patients. Children still sat on verandas and played in the sand, and one former nurse recalled that in the late twentieth century the staff continued to bring children to the ocean and chat "about the therapeutic importance of salt water" as they watched their charges swim.[84] But doctors no longer prescribed marine medication's programmatic sea air, seawater, and sunbathing practices; neither Howard nor Edward described experiences that sounded like the seashore therapies that physicians supported in earlier decades. While place-based therapeutics had receded with the tides of time, pleasure and play remained important elements of Americans' perceptions of the seashore's identity. Children's time at the beach helped shape Americans' notions of the seashore as a tourist attraction and vacation destination for families.

SIX DOCTOR SUN AND TECHNOLOGIES OF NATURE

MARINE MEDICATION is no longer part of medical practice. Yet, neither doctors nor the public outright rejected the notion that the beach could cure. Knowing this begs the question: how and why did we lose our medical conceptualization of the seashore as a therapeutic landscape?

Images in the Boston Floating Hospital's 1925 annual report suggest an answer. A photograph shows a tall, lean man dressed in a tie and a physician's customary long white coat. He wears a pair of tinted goggles as he adjusts a bulky UV lamp above a bare-chested toddler, who lies in a drop-side crib. The child bends one arm above its head and gazes through begoggled eyes at the wall. A nurse monitors the child, her vision unencumbered by protective eyewear. The caption explains that Dr. Lawrence Smith is treating a patient who has rickets.[1]

This photograph is a dramatic departure from others images the hospital circulated just a few decades earlier. In the late nineteenth and early twentieth centuries, the hospital promoted its grand white ship floating in Boston's harbor. Crowds of mothers and babies clustered on the decks, milling among the medical staff. Hammocks gently rocked resting children. On the sundeck, naked toddlers lined up along the railing. Some of the children have rickets' tell-tale bowed legs. Gazing at the water, the children, with their bodies bare, bathe in the natural sunlight.

Juxtaposing the two photographs of children receiving light treatment for rickets implies that technologies, including UV lamps, replaced environmental therapeutics. It is a tidy historical trajectory that aligns with well-documented transformations of American health care. Historians have traced the infiltration of machines into clinical encounters. Sphygmomanometers and

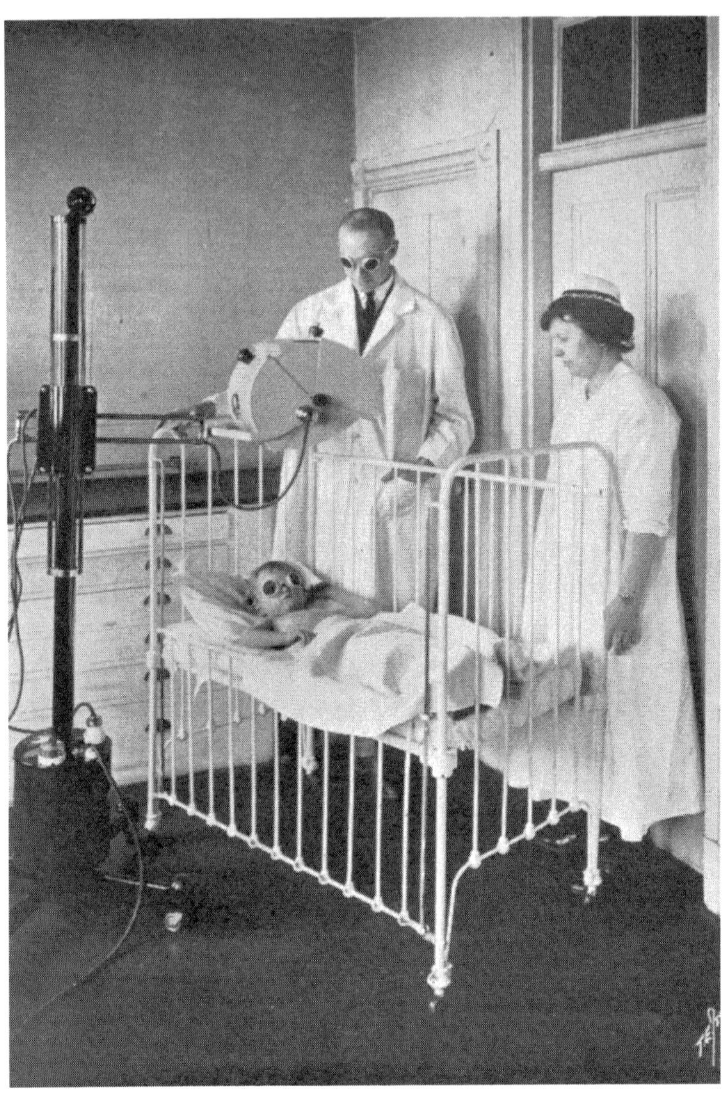

FIGURE 17. Child undergoing UV lamp treatment for rickets at the Boston Floating Hospital, 1925. Boston Floating Hospital, *Thirty-Second Annual Report*, 1925, 32–33. Courtesy of Countway Library, Harvard University.

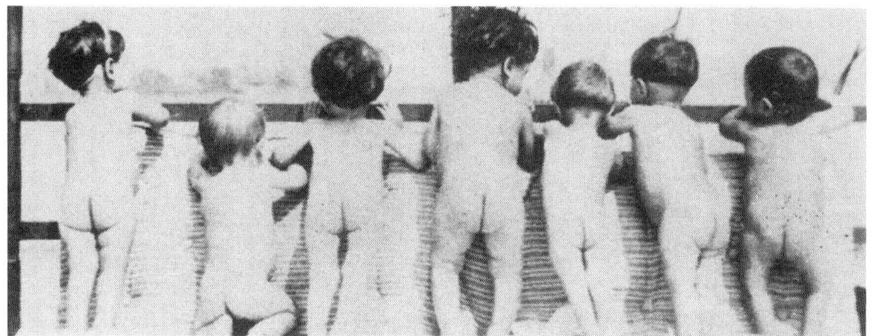

FIGURE 18. "Toddlers on the Boston Floating Hospital ship's sundeck." This image from the early twentieth century shows young children receiving natural sunlight therapy. New England Medical Center Records, http://hdl.handle.net/10427/004942. ID: 4m90f390b.

stethoscopes, x-rays and autoclaves, vaccines and antitoxin had been added to physicians' technological arsenal by the early twentieth century.[2] Urban hospitals housed many of these technologies, and patients became accustomed to their use within institutional settings. It is logical to conclude that physicians and nurses would easily swap sunbathing for a sun lamp.

This transition did not immediately occur. In the early twentieth century, American physicians and patients largely rejected the UV lamps in favor of natural sunbathing. It was surprising to learn that UV lamps predated "heliotherapy," the systematized practice of natural sunbathing. In the early twentieth century, many American physicians even warned colleagues against using the devices, claiming that technologies could not approximate what nature provided.[3]

This chapter argues that the eventual adoption of sunlamps did not signify a medical rejection of environmental therapeutics, including marine medication. It instead reflected a simultaneous belief in nature's curative effects and the necessity of treating patients in cities. We will see how American physicians initially rejected artificial light treatment for both pragmatic and ideological reasons and that UV lamps were not the result of a belief in technological superiority. Rather, the devices were born from the scientific knowledge that natural sunlight could cure. American practitioners only fully adopted technologies once they replicated natural sunlight's outcomes and thereby helped doctors overcome the environmental limitations of urban medical practice.

Over the twentieth century doctors and scientists used scientific knowledge to build machines that mimicked sunlight's therapeutic and preventive effects.[4] It took them some time, but, once achieved, it was no longer necessary to prescribe a trip outside of the city. Technologies like UV lamps increasingly displaced environmental interventions. As a result, it became harder to look at spaces like the seashore as a therapeutic landscape or to understand that UV lamps project a faith that nature can cure.

Heliotherapy: Natural Therapeutics in the Age of Scientific Medicine

In the early twentieth century, boosters celebrated the abundant and health-giving rays at America's beaches, and seashore hospitals included sunbathing as part of their medical regimens. Both Sea Breeze in New York and the Children's Seashore House in Atlantic City published pictures of patients sunbathing on the sand and lying on verandas and sundecks for their dose of sunlight. Time outdoors had always been an important aspect of marine medication, and by the 1910s there had been a slight but important shift. Physicians started to advocate for and implement "heliotherapy." Auguste Rollier had pioneered the method at his mountaintop sanatorium in Europe. His primary invention was a standardized dosing of natural sunlight through graduated exposure.

As noted in chapter 2, heliotherapy began with exposing patients' feet, followed by their shins, legs, and then torso over a series of days. Practitioners considered tanned skin a sign that the treatment was working. Once a patient's skin was fully pigmented, medical practitioners allowed patients to sunbathe for three hours a day.[5] This intervention often required venturing outdoors, even in the snow, wearing little more than a loincloth.[6]

By 1910, John Brannan, a physician affiliated with Sea Breeze, had become aware of Rollier's work through American and French colleagues. Brannan was impressed by heliotherapy's results, and in 1912 Sea Breeze implemented Rollier's program.[7] Brannan reported that patients with long-standing sinuses had shown "rapid improvement" after heliotherapy and that "in almost all cases the general condition is apparently much benefited."[8] He acknowledged that nurses had attributed the "favourable effect of the sea water on sinuses and skin lesions, and I have now no doubt that the sun's rays played a large part in the healing process."[9] Crawford Allen Hospital in Rhode Island also adopted versions of Rollier's sunbathing regimen. Heliotherapy's standardized natural sun exposure made it a good fit with both the rationalized and natural therapeutics programs already employed at seashore hospitals.[10]

Heliotherapy advocates celebrated the myriad benefits natural sunbathing provided. Physicians documented how recalcitrant wounds suddenly healed, patients' metabolisms spiked, and hemoglobin soared. Practitioners heralded these changes as laboratory evidence that the sun increased blood's bactericidal properties and shielded patients against the intrusion of disease.[11] They also documented that sunbathing "stimulates the recalcification of the entire bony skeleton," thereby strengthening and straightening pediatric patients' bones.[12]

Photographs captured patients' incredible physical transformations, offering visual evidence of the sunlight treatment's success. Rollier published a multitude of photographs that displayed patients' progressions from sickness to health.[13] Images, including x-rays, documented that doses of sunlight cured disease, healed bones, and reformed bodies. Marine medication practitioners also employed photographs as proof of the sun's healing properties. In 1921, Henry Gauvain documented his tubercular patients' recoveries. One image from the Hayling Island care facility showed patients undergoing heliotherapy while gardening. Even though all ten patients suffered from tuberculosis, abscesses, and/or sinuses, they worked the soil, most without the aid of crutches or other devices. Gauvain instructed his colleagues to "note the excellent condition and muscular development."[14]

Gauvain further supported the seashore's salutary effects with a series of three photographs of a patient at the seaside hospital on Hayling Island. The text explained that the patient had pulmonary tuberculosis that resulted in "cranial caries, cervical adenitis, tuberculous disease of both elbows, both wrists, both hips, both knees, both ankles, severe mesenteric tubercle with threatened intestinal obstruction; numerous abscesses and sinuses."[15] The accompanying photographs document the patients' dire condition and

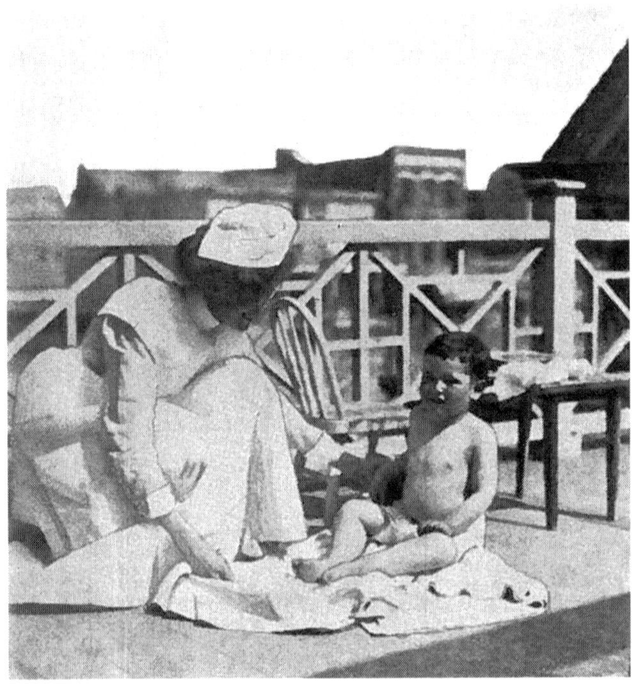

FIGURE 19. Child undergoing heliotherapy at Sea Breeze Hospital. In Guy Hinsdale, *Atmospheric Air in Relation to Tuberculosis* (Washington, DC: Smithsonian Institution, 1914), plate 15.

subsequent transformation. In the first image the child looks sullenly at the camera; her swollen joints protrude from her skeletal frame. She lies on her back, so weak that an attendant props up her frail, misshapen arm for the photographer. The girl is pale, emaciated, and appears to be at death's door. The following image shows a remarkable change. A bather holds the girl while she floats in the ocean. Despite needing assistance to submerge in the water, the girl's cheeks appear fuller as she looks happily toward the shore.

The final photograph displays further evidence of the treatment's efficacy. The girl stands unassisted, with her right leg only slightly turned inward and significant weight gain evident to viewers. Sporting a big bow in her hair and tan lines from the splint she has worn, the girl proudly stands, with a wide smile completing the picture of physical health.[16]

By focusing their cameras on patients, physicians documented that heliotherapy, alongside other seaside therapeutics, resulted in physical transformations. Photographic evidence of patients' newly straightened spines, mobile joints, healed sinuses, and sturdy bodies confirmed that sunlight and other environmental elements could cure.[17] When tourists visited seashore hospitals, they witnessed bed-bound patients sleeping outdoors on hospital porches, while other children frolicked on the beach in the sun and sea air. The scenes suggest that the sun facilitated the youths' progression from bedridden to healthy and able-bodied.

At once scientific and natural, heliotherapy fit into existing institutional structures at seashore hospitals, including long-standing environmental therapeutic practices. It also built upon ideas about children's connectivity with and need for healthy outdoor spaces. Heliotherapy's systematic approach to dosing also aligned with the trend toward more quantitatively, data-driven medical practices.

Once at the seashore, or on a mountaintop, sunlight could cure children of disease, but sending every urban patient with rickets or nonpulmonary tuberculosis to the seashore was not pragmatic. Moreover, the medical milieu had already shifted by the time Americans had begun to adopt heliotherapeutics. In 1914, Brannan lamented that he found it "almost impossible to interest surgeons or physicians" in practicing "heliotherapy or any form of outdoor treatment."[18] Empirical evidence such as healed wounds and before and after photographs was not enough to compel most physicians to adopt heliotherapy. By the 1920s, the advancement of UV lights was further contributing to reluctance by making it easier to administer healthy doses of sunlight, even under polluted city skies and in interior urban hospital rooms.

UV Lamps: Projecting Sunlight's Therapeutic Benefits

While at first children at American seashore hospitals received heliotherapy outdoors, patients at some European institutions knew both technological and natural sunlight treatments. British doctors heralded the sun for its curative potential for children with diseases such as tuberculosis and rickets, but physicians at pediatric seashore hospitals also knew they could not count on the sun to break through cloud cover or to shine brightly enough to produce results.[19] They turned to UV lamps to fill the void left by the dark skies in their northern latitude.[20]

Even physicians' adoption of UV lamps reflected their conviction that sunlight could cure. Scientific evidence increasingly supported the sun's potential to produce therapeutic results. In the same decade that the Children's Seashore House opened in Atlantic City, British physician Arthur Downes and chemist Thomas Blunt identified the sun's bactericidal properties. They studied sunlight's effects on bacteria and fungi, concluding that sunlight stunted the development of both. They also determined that the actinic (UV) rays killed bacteria.[21] After Robert Koch identified the tubercle bacillus in 1882, physicians realized the therapeutic potential of Downes and Blunt's finding, positing that, if sunlight was bactericidal, it could treat diseases like tuberculosis.

Some physicians, including Rollier, applied this knowledge to support natural sunbathing. Others used it as inspiration to build devices that mimicked the sun's UV rays. This latter group included Niels Finsen, a physician practicing in Denmark, who in the 1890s invented the first UV lamp. As with Downes and Blunt, Finsen had conducted a range of experiments that solidified his beliefs in the sun's therapeutic value. His investigations demonstrated that sun exposure resulted in the skin's darkening and that pigmentation protected skin from burning. He also discovered that sunlight could penetrate skin and that UV exposure enhanced animals' development.[22]

When Finsen first started to care for patients, he applied this knowledge and included natural sunbathing as part of their treatment. Patients would lie on a cot outdoors while a nurse manipulated a large lens to concentrate the sun's rays onto a specific portion of the patient's skin. Finsen abandoned this method after finding it too difficult to "rely on sunlight in northern latitudes."[23] The sunshine in Denmark simply was not strong or consistent enough.

Environmental constraints led Finsen to develop a lamp that could produce UV rays strong enough to cure patients of tuberculosis. He proved his lamps' utility when he successfully treated his first patient, a man who had suffered from skin tuberculosis for eight years. Artificial UV therapy cured the patient within four months. Word spread and patients flocked from around the world for Finsen's artificial UV light treatment. One physician labeled Copenhagen a "mecca" for skin tuberculosis patients.[24] The UV lamps' successes even won notice with the Nobel Prize Committee.[25] The committee awarded Finsen the Nobel Prize in Physiology or Medicine in 1903, "in recognition of his contribution to the treatment of diseases, especially lupus vulgaris, with concentrated light radiation, whereby he has opened a new avenue for medical science."[26]

American physicians were initially less sanguine about UV lamps. Physicians balked at them for many reasons. They complained that early lamps were too big and expensive and that their operation required a highly trained staff.[27] The lamp required electric current that could cost upwards of $3,000 per year, the equivalent of more than $100,000 today. In 1903, American orthopedic surgeon DeForest Willard, a marine medication supporter, decried this as a "serious" expenditure.[28] The operating requirements for early UV lamps forced at least one New York physician to wire the unit directly to the power lines outside his office and another physician to abandon its installation altogether.[29]

Early UV lights were also cumbersome. The Finsen lamp was a hulking device, consisting of four arms that extended at 45-degree angles from a central lamp. It weighed so much it required iron supports to suspend it from the ceiling. The arms consisted of two adjustable brass tubes, with one telescoping into the other. Two lenses at the top of the wider tube gathered the lamp's rays, which then traveled down the arms to a second set of lenses that concentrated and focused the light. Cooled, distilled water had to continuously flow between the second set of lenses to absorb the rays' heat and thereby protect patients' skin from burning. At the tip of each arm was another lens that nurses placed firmly against patients' skin.[30]

Photographs documented that early UV lamps required a skilled nurse to attend to one patient at a time. Nurses had to maneuver and focus the UV lamp directly over the region that required treatment. Patients would lie beneath the lamp for up to two hours while nurses tended to patients' needs. At the end of treatment, nurses applied a zinc ointment on the patient's skin to facilitate healing. Patients receiving care at Finsen's institute would leave the facility only to return for more treatment the following day. This process continued for months, stopping only once the patient healed.[31]

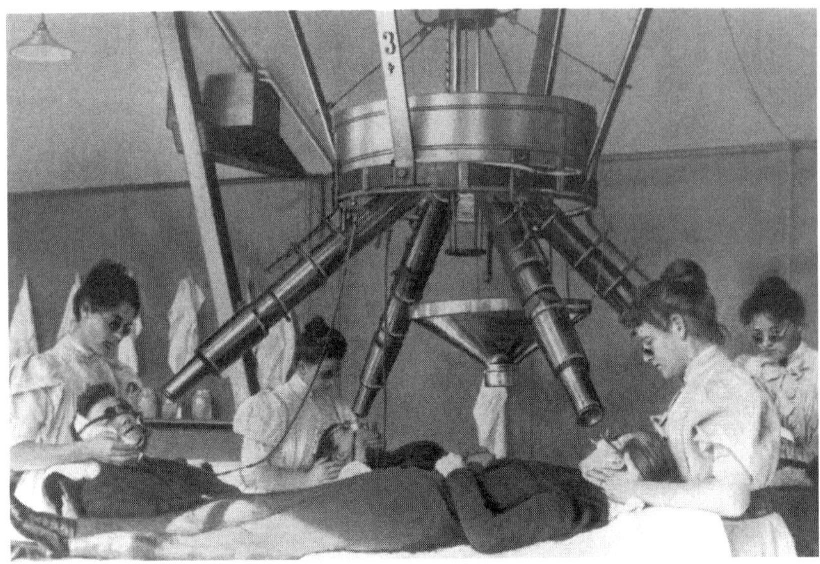

FIGURE 20. Niels Finsen's UV lamp, 1900. Note the size of the structure and the one-on-one care that nurses provide to patients during treatment. Signal Photos/Alamy Stock Photo.

American physicians also initially believed that natural sunlight yielded superior results. New York physician W. S. Gottheil attempted to use an "American form of the Finsen apparatus" but concluded he could achieve similar outcomes through easier methods.[32] In 1907, physician Jay Frank Schamberg postulated that the Finsen Institute's relative success in treating skin tuberculosis was the result of their staff's expertise, writing, "In the light institute of Copenhagen . . . better results are obtained than elsewhere by reason of the skill of the physicians and the experience of the nurses."[33] In 1903, Willard outlined his belief in the superiority of natural sunlight therapy in the treatment of patients with bone and joint tuberculosis. In an article published in the *Journal of the American Medical Association*, he argued that "the most powerful agents in our possession for the inhibition and destruction of these micro-organisms are sunlight and fresh air and abundant nourishment. The sun's rays are undoubtedly more helpful than any artificial rays, just as natural waters compounded by the chemistry of the Ruler of the universe differ very decidedly from the waters artificially compounded by the chemistry of man."[34] Willard's statement underscores his conviction that naturally available resources therapeutically surpassed technological approximations.

Yet from the beginning it was clear that UV lamps could be effective, if light doses were administered correctly. As with heliotherapy, photographic evidence was proof that UV therapy worked, producing curative and positive cosmetic effects.[35] For instance, a thirty-year-old patient treated at Finsen's Institute had facial and nasal skin tuberculosis for fifteen years. When the woman arrived for light therapy, she had an extensive area of red, swollen, diseased skin that stretched across both cheeks, her nose, and her upper lip. She also had numerous nodules and small ulcerations and crusts in the diseased skin. After four months of treatment, the patient's ulcers were gone, she had fewer nodules, and her facial skin and nose appeared healthy, with "good scar tissue" forming. By the end of the fifth month, the patient's remaining nodules had disappeared, and her treatment was complete. One year later, the patient's doctor reported that she was still healthy and had suffered no relapse.[36]

By the 1920s, scientists were equating the outcomes from natural and artificial sunbathing. In 1926, physician W. Kerr Russell wrote to the *British Medical Journal* to compare results between patients treated by UV lamps at Finsen's Institute and heliotherapy patients' outcomes at Rollier's sanatorium. Russell concluded that patients' results at the two institutions were "almost identical. . . . In a few cases the Finsen results are even better than those obtained at Leysin," the Swiss village where Rollier's clinic was located. Russell acknowledged that "natural sun treatment has certain advantages in the prevention and cure of disease," but he maintained that heliotherapy's benefits depended on the environmental and geographical context. He claimed that it was "impossible to practice heliotherapy satisfactorily in the North of England in the winter; even . . . by the use of 'vita-glass,' my great standby has been ultra-violet lamps."[37] Russell did not deny heliotherapy's results but qualified them as specific to certain places. He further concluded that "it cannot seriously be suggested that it is possible or desirable to send all tuberculous patients to Switzerland."[38] Practitioners in the United States started to embrace the same logic and slowly added UV lamps to their therapeutic tool kit.

Moving toward the Light

American physicians maintained their practices of marine medication and natural sun exposure well into the twentieth century, but the number of pediatric patients in cities only grew. Physicians looked for solutions closer to home to treat the swelling number of children who might benefit from sun exposure. They identified children with rickets as particularly good candidates for UV light therapy.[39] New diagnostic tools such as x-rays (1895) revealed that the disease was far more widespread than previously recognized. Around the turn of the century physicians had determined that up to 90 percent of children suffered from rickets.[40] Scientists continued to believe that the disease was due to a lack of sun exposure, and it made sense to conclude that spending time outside, under the sun, would buffer children from developing rickets. Physicians tested their hypothesis by providing programs of sun exposure and discovered that UV rays cured and prevented rickets.

There was a pressing need to care for nearly every urban child, but American physicians did not quickly adopt artificial light therapies. This was true despite German investigators who claimed "astonishingly favorable results" when using artificial light for treating rickets. Renowned American physicians and rickets experts Alfred Hess and Lester Unger remained skeptical. As late as 1921 they concluded that UV lamps neither prevented nor treated rickets. They insisted that "[ultra]violet ray treatment cannot be considered equivalent to heliotherapy."[41]

Within a year Hess and Unger amended their claim. In 1922, they published an article in the *Journal of the American Medical Association* contending that carbon arc lamps had "been found, in the laboratory as well as in the clinic, to be a very effective therapeutic agent in the prevention and cure of rickets."[42] Hess and Unger did not deny that heliotherapy also worked. In fact, they began their article by reminding readers that "attention has been called to the curative effect of sunlight in infantile rickets." Moreover, they decided to study a carbon arc lamp because its light more "nearly approaches the sun's spectrum" when compared to other lamps.[43] This decision underscores their faith in sunlight's therapeutic value, even as it became encapsulated within a device. UV lamps and heliotherapy together helped institute sunbathing as a medical and social practice in the 1920s, with technological cures placed alongside environmental interventions.

At the same time Hess, Unger, and others were studying UV light treatment, scientists and physicians were looking for additional technological treatments. Other colleagues had postulated that rickets was caused by a nutritional deficiency. They had induced rickets in rats and dogs by limiting their diets and then curing them with certain foods, including cod liver oil and milk. These scientists hypothesized that lack of a form of vitamin A resulted in rickets. By 1922, they had refined their protocols and determined that deficiency of a yet-unidentified vitamin was the culprit. They named this substance vitamin D.[44]

Soon thereafter, Harriette Chick, a bacteriologist and researcher at the University of Vienna, found that both cod liver oil and sunlight exposure cured rickets. She determined that a combination of the two interventions resulted in faster recovery time and that children who were treated in outdoor settings showed more rapid general improvement than those remaining in the wards.[45] Two years later, University of Wisconsin biochemistry professor Harry Steenbock promoted fortifying food with vitamin D to cure and prevent the disease. Supplemented cereals and milk offered a more palatable solution than the foul-tasting cod liver oil.[46]

Nutritional supplements and UV lamps provided technological interventions to cure what physicians had labeled an environmentally induced disease.[47] By the mid-1920s, other scientists had confirmed Hess and Unger's finding, concluding that artificial and natural light produced changes in blood chemistry similar to other antirachitic substances, such as vitamin D–rich foods.[48] By 1930, American scientists were claiming that it was "well known" that ultraviolet rays from mercury vapor arc lamps could be used in the "prevention and cure of rickets."[49] Hospitals across the United States and Europe could flip a switch and treat large groups of patients indoors, in city centers, while mothers in their homes served children bowls of fortified cereals with irradiated milk.

Although physicians adopted new technologies, they did not reject natural sunlight as a beneficial therapy. This belief even led urban hospitals to attempt to integrate heliotherapy into their treatment programs. Institutions modified porches and roofs into "solariums," and in 1927 a nurse at New Haven Hospital in Connecticut designed a heliotherapy tent to protect patients' privacy from onlookers.[50] However, in a way reminiscent of Finsen's complaints, urban physicians lamented the difficulty of accessing enough sunlight in the city to make heliotherapy effective. As Cincinnati physician R. Plato Schwartz explained, cloudy days and the varying intensity of the sun made for "less favorable results from the use of heliotherapy when attempted in the modern city hospital."[51]

The promise of heliotherapy continued to draw patients and physicians from the city to the seashore well into the twentieth century. In the early 1930s, famed architect Cass Gilbert designed the Seaside Sanatorium in Waterford, Connecticut, along Long Island Sound, for the "heliotropic" treatment of tubercular children.[52] Physicians remained open to environmental treatments, even while embracing technological interventions.

Back in the cities, where skyscrapers and pollution blocked the sunlight, health care professionals turned to artificial light sources. Frederick Tisdall, a physician at the Hospital for Sick Children in Toronto, noted that the therapeutic rays of the sun were "readily cut off by the smoke[,] dust and moisture" in the unclean air of industrial cities. Given the lack of statistics for North America, Tisdall pointed to a comparative study of the strength of UV rays in London, the British countryside, and the Swiss Alps and concluded that London's pollution lowered the intensity of the UV rays by 85 percent relative to conditions on Switzerland's mountaintops.[53]

UV lamps became increasingly appealing as newer devices remedied many of the concerns that American physicians had registered with earlier designs. By the 1920s, the devices had become smaller and easier to use, and they required fewer attendants to operate them. They consumed less energy, making them cheaper to run. The lamps allowed doctors to administer the therapeutic properties of the sun without having to worry about the weather or latitude. When urban hospitals provided access to UV lamps, they enabled patients to receive treatment closer to home, a solution that benefited doctors and the families they treated.[54] Moreover, instead of treating only four patients at a time, like Finsen's model, newer lamps could treat dozens of children simultaneously.

In the mid-1920s, R. Plato Schwartz detailed Cincinnati General Hospital's use of a UV light that could treat twenty to thirty patients at once.[55] Even very young children received treatment in groups. One photograph reproduced in multiple texts shows five toddlers in a playpen. The children wore diapers and protective goggles while receiving UV light therapy from several lamps.[56] Other images show children gathered around sunlamps, with their hands raised as if worshipping the light.[57] The images and accompanying descriptions of UV light therapy suggest that the technologies were simple to use and did not require the same degree of oversight as earlier models. Images depict only a few, if any, medical attendants overseeing the therapy.

Just as critically, by the 1920s scientists had created lamps that more closely mimicked the sun's rays. In 1926, Schwartz celebrated that his midwestern hospital's lamps produced a spectrum of light wherein the "therapeutic reactions are practically identical to those obtained by exposure to sunlight." He explained that "it seems safe to state that it is no longer necessary to depend upon the sun which produces radiant energy of known therapeutic value in the treatment of chronic diseases, and there is some justification for believing that an exact reproduction of sunlight will ultimately be obtained by further improvements in the lamp which is now in operation."[58] Schwartz linguistically melded nature and technology. His equation of "improvement" with an "exact reproduction of sunlight" indicates that he saw reproducing natural sunlight as the goal. Even as physicians, including Schwartz, Hess, and Unger, embraced UV lamps, they upheld the sun's ability to heal.

The ability to artificially produce sunlight meant that physicians had overcome the limitations of their environments. Once they captured nature's curative capabilities within a device, practitioners could provide patients with the benefits of the sun, regardless of latitude, weather, pollution, or skyscrapers. With proof that artificial lights produced the same outcomes as natural sunlight, physicians melded technology and nature.

Homegrown: Children under the Sun

As physicians incorporated UV lamps into their practice, they handed off the administration of natural sunbathing to mothers and children.[59] The

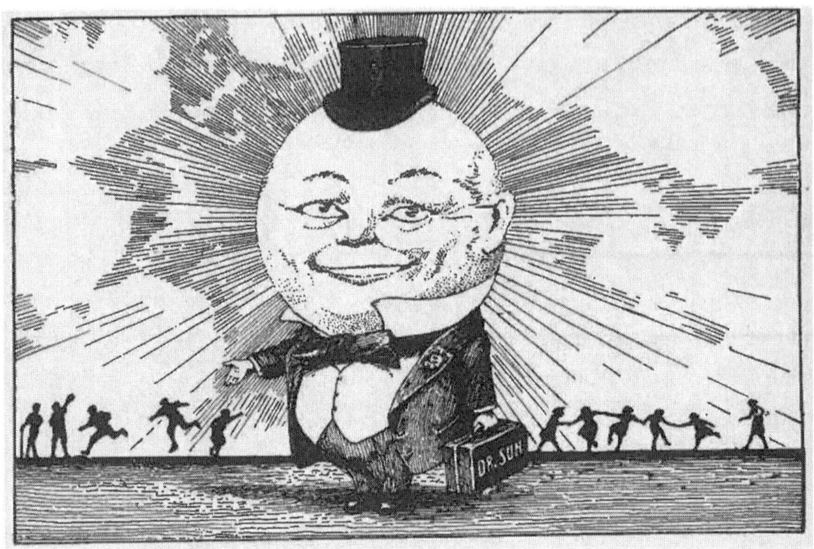

FIGURE 21. "Our Friend the Sun." In this drawing, included in a health textbook for children, "Dr. Sun" beams, motioning toward children as if taking credit for their healthy play. J. Mace Andress and W. A. Evans, *Health and Success* (Boston: Ginn and Company, 1925), 117.

decoupling of heliotherapy from medical practitioners further distanced physicians from environmental therapeutics.

In 1925, J. Mace Andress, a lecturer on health education, and W. A. Evans, a physician and former president of the American Public Health Association, published *Health and Success*, a textbook for children. In the chapter "Our Friend the Sun," the sun appears as a physician wearing a suit and top hat and carrying a bag inscribed "Dr. Sun." The glowing orb smiles as he extends his arm to the silhouettes of children running and playing behind him, as if claiming credit for their health and happiness.[60] The chapter informs its young readers that "sunshine, good air, and good food are all necessary for health" and that children need the sun to become healthy, "rosy-cheeked" individuals.[61]

Young readers learned that the sun could cure diseases. The authors taught them that "in days of old, children often had a disease which was called 'the king's evil.' One reason why it was called by that name was that people believed a touch of the king's hand would cure it."[62] They explained that physicians renamed the king's evil, calling it "scrofula," or tuberculosis of the glands. By the 1920s, people no longer believed that a king could cure the disease. Yet children read that "in a sense it is 'the king's evil,' but the king is the sun. Those who do not get enough sunlight are liable to have this disease. The touch of King Sun cures it. He is one of the world's best friends."[63] Sunlight was not only beneficial for children with scrofula but was also "excellent for sick children. . . . It has been found that children who are very ill because of weak lungs or rickets may be cured by letting the sunshine in upon them."[64]

Physicians and scientists relied on analogies to explain sunlight's impact on bodies and growth. Andress and Evans asked children to think about potatoes they might find in a cellar. Such potatoes may have sprouts or even leaves, the authors wrote, but the plants are "very pale and unhealthy looking, very different from the green potato plants which grow out of doors in the sunlight."[65] The authors told children that kids who "live in dark houses and spend little time in playing in the fresh air and sunshine are likely to be pale and unhealthy like the potatoes that grow in a cellar."[66]

The authors built their lessons on the latest medical and public health knowledge. Just one year later, Toronto physician R. I. Harris wrote, "Plants deprived of sunlight grow up pale, weak and spindly; so do children. Plants grown in sunlight become deeply colored[,] sturdy and strong. . . . In children the same analogy holds." Like many public health officials, Harris believed that tanning could prevent or cure rickets and that sunlight positively affected children's bone growth and development. He additionally hypothesized that sunlight could treat Pott's disease (tuberculosis of the spine and joints), writing, "It may well be that this action of sun upon skeletal tissues explains its almost specific effect upon tuberculosis of bones and joints."[67]

Health professionals shared their knowledge of sunlight's curative potential with children and their mothers. Likewise, popular periodicals, such as *Good Housekeeping*, published articles that targeted women and mothers to teach them about the benefits of sunlight.[68] While some texts acknowledged the impact of sun on different skin tones, authors primarily addressed children with light skin tones.

Doctors and public health officials promoted tanning, as did the US Children's Bureau. Its 1926 pamphlet *Sunlight for Babies*, the US Children's Bureau highlighted the benefits of sunbathing. The circular warned, "If a baby is constantly deprived of direct sunlight his bones will not develop normally, his muscles will be flabby, and his skin will be pale. He will probably have rickets."[69] To prevent this fate, the bureau encouraged mothers to begin sunbaths when infants were three or four weeks old. Mothers learned how to gradually expose their babies to the sun, to tan rather than burn the skin, and that "a good tan is evidence that the ultra-violet rays are being effective."[70]

While the recommendation for tanning is at odds twenty-first-century teaching, at the time it represented elite medical knowledge. It also corresponded to cultural shifts regarding sun exposure. During the nineteenth century, people regarded a pale visage as a sign of elite social status and beauty. Many Americans lived and worked on farms, and therefore a tanned face indicated one's outdoor labor. Only people with means could maintain pale skin.[71] As the United States began to industrialize and the working classes moved indoors, pallid faces provided evidence of a life spent working inside.

Concurrently, cultural elites' definition of beauty shifted from a porcelain complexion to rosy cheeks. Tanned skin became a marker of the ability to afford leisure time and access to a sunny climate. As health and leisure became intertwined during this period, so too did the association of a tanned skin with health. *Sunlight for Babies* aligned with these trends. The pamphlet informed mothers that "tanning is the goal for which to strive."[72] Mothers received the message. In 1930, *Sunlight for Babies* was the Children's Bureau's second most popular pamphlet (*Why Sleep* was first), with a distribution of more than sixty-three thousand copies in a single year.[73]

The movement of heliotherapy into the home was in line with maternal responsibilities for scientific child rearing. In the early twentieth century mothers sought advice from medical professionals and government officials regarding how to best care for their children.[74] Physicians taught mothers that children's bodies were plastic and could be reformed through environmental changes.[75] Women learned that children's physical malleability enabled babies to overcome diseases if given access to the sun and fresh air. Health experts and social reformers expressed concern that ill children would "swell the ever-growing numbers of that pitiable mass of humanity, the useless and the unfit."[76] Sunlight could change that course, and mothers oversaw the intervention.

Mothers received instruction for at-home heliotherapy. The US Children's Bureau provided women with specific time and exposure recommendations, according to season and geographical location. Mothers learned that springtime babies should begin outdoor sunbathing in March or April, or earlier for families who lived in the South. During the first bath mothers "let the sun shine on his face and hands for 10 to 15 minutes, with his cap pushed back or taken off." From there mothers needed to "each day lengthen the time—by 3 minutes for a fair baby and by 5 minutes for a dark baby. After the face and hands are used to exposure, roll up the sleeves. Soon the stockings may be taken off; then the dress, shirt and band. After a month or two the baby should be getting half an hour of sun in the morning and half an hour in the afternoon, wearing only a diaper."[77] The gradual exposure of more surface area for greater lengths of time, with the objective of ultimately wearing only a diaper, derives from Rollier's system of sunlight exposure.

As heliotherapy shifted from the hospital to the home, it was transformed from a medical to a domestic practice. Its relative simplicity meant that anyone could oversee its application. UV lamps, in contrast, maintained their medical associations. Although some manufacturers marketed UV lamps to the general public, the officials at the US Children's Bureau cautioned mothers to consult their physicians before using the devices.[78]

When physicians handed off heliotherapy to mothers, that transfer did not indicate that medical practitioners rejected its efficacy. Rather, like thermometers or aspirin, natural sunbathing did not require medical expertise or professional oversight.[79] With this shift, physicians distanced themselves from nature-based interventions even as they simultaneously embraced their technological counterparts.

THE PHOTOGRAPHS included near the beginning of this chapter hint at larger transitions to come but don't capture the nuanced change over time. When Dr. Lawrence Smith oversaw UV light therapy inside the Boston Floating Hospital in 1925, he used a technology that projected a faith that nature could cure. Sunlight remained a crucial therapeutic tool, but it could now be accessed indoors, under a lamp.

The magnitude of this shift toward technological solutions is captured by the Boston Floating Hospital's move from a ship to a landlocked hospital building. In 1927, a fire destroyed the once grand hospital ship. Faced with the decision about how to best care for its pediatric patients, the hospital's officials determined that they could rebuild the hospital in Boston's center. By 1930, physicians could justify moving their patients from outdoor porches and sundecks that overlooked the ocean to interior hospital rooms located in dense urban settings.[80] Technologies like the UV lamp reflected large-scale changes in the United States and Europe. As urban populations swelled, hospitals struggled to keep up with demand. New devices, based on the latest, laboratory-based science, promised to treat and even cure more patients, with greater control, closer to home. Once technologies mimicked environmental elements, technologies such as UV lamps freed natural therapeutics from the constraints of place. As a result, it became harder to look at the beach and see it as a necessary site for medical care.

UV lamps have scientific origins in a belief that nature can cure. But looking at them today, the devices do not conjure an association of the sun glinting off the ocean or warming children at play on the beach. The same may hold true for other technologies that derive from environmental therapeutics. Bags of saline solution hanging from metal poles hardly evoke the feeling of ocean waves as they crest and break over adults and children enjoying a day at the beach, yet medical articles from the early twentieth century suggest a direct lineage.[81] Likewise, the hum of air conditioners does not trigger the sensation of ocean breezes coming through large windows. Sunlight and salt water have remained medically efficacious, but their evolution into technologies of nature has made the environmental connections essentially invisible.

CONCLUSION

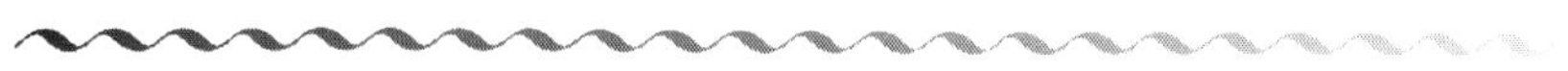

IN 2006, CNN REPORTED that physician Scott Donaldson had made an exciting discovery: seawater was an effective treatment for patients with cystic fibrosis (CF). Donaldson, who practiced in North Carolina, realized that his patients who surfed had fewer lung exacerbations than patients who did not take to the waves. This realization was significant because CF causes mucus buildup and infections in the lungs, which inhibits patients' breathing and can lead to hospitalization.[1] Donaldson wondered if there "might be something about saltwater that could explain improved lung function in the surfers."[2]

To test this hypothesis, Donaldson conducted randomized controlled trials to determine if saline exposure improved patients' outcomes. Donaldson and his colleague, William Bennett, enrolled patients and administered either a 7 percent saline solution, a 7 percent saline solution with a pretreatment of amiloride (a drug intended to increase saline solution's effects), or a 0.9 percent saline solution. They hypothesized that the amiloride group would outperform the 7 percent saline-only group. To their surprise, they discovered that saline alone provided patients with the most substantial clinical benefits, including an improved ability to clear mucus and lower rates of hospitalization. Amiloride negated the advantage.[3] The authors published their results in the *New England Journal of Medicine*, concluding that inhaling hypertonic saline solution that was preceded by a bronchodilator was "an inexpensive, safe, and effective additional therapy for patients."[4]

Donaldson was "blown away" by the results. The idea that something as inexpensive and abundant as seawater could reduce hospitalizations by half and "significantly [improve a patient's] ability to clear mucus from the lungs" shocked him. A reporter crowed, "An effective treatment has long been elusive, and now it seems that one was hiding in plain sight: in the world's oceans."[5]

Despite these findings, twenty-first-century physicians did not start prescribing time at the seashore to their patients, nor did Donaldson mention either the beach or surfing in his *New England Journal of Medicine* article. Rather, medical professionals learned that patients inhaled saline through a nebulizer, a device that delivers medication via mist.

Five years later in Los Angeles, a father named Mark Smith read a new medical journal article that reported the benefits of saltwater mist for infants and toddlers with cystic fibrosis.[6] Smith's three-year-old daughter, Mallory, had just been diagnosed with CF. Learning about the benefits of exposure to sea air, Mark and his wife, Diane, made the beach the center of their daughter's life. For Mallory Smith, whose posthumous memoir *Salt in My Soul: An Unfinished Life* (2019) chronicles her relationship to cystic fibrosis and the ocean, the seashore was a space of respite where she could breathe easier and pursue her passion of surfing.

Mallory's use of the seashore reflected the practices of families from a century earlier, while Donaldson's surprise highlights how much had changed over time. Reductionist trends, coupled with the rise of laboratory-based medicine and randomized controlled trials, have made it difficult to advocate for environmental interventions as medical treatments.[7] Physicians might recognize the connections, but professional standards elevate laboratory-based forms of evidence and relegate environmental observations to the background. Doctors had once rushed to write prescriptions for patients to spend time at the beach.[8] Yet, even a century later, for children like Mallory the natural world held the promise of health.

Donaldson, like many medical practitioners before him, never rejected the idea that exposure to nature could be healthy. Instead, as this book has shown, a series of forces altered Americans' ways of knowing, seeing, and experiencing their bodies at the beach. Shifts in medical knowledge production, as well as the rise of leisure culture, gradually obscured Americans' conceptualizations of the interconnections between the environment and human health.

This book has charted the retreat from environmental explanations of health and examined how tourists consumed and altered cultural associations of the beach. Practices that began in the late nineteenth century accelerated throughout the twentieth century. By the 1930s, both children and adults could access new vaccines and lifesaving medications. Newspapers told heroic stories of lifesaving drugs, such as when teams of dogsleds dashed over frozen tundra to procure antiserum that saved children in Nome, Alaska, from the grip of a diphtheria outbreak. New treatments transformed diseases from fatal ailments to chronic conditions.[9] The mass production of penicillin in the 1940s cured bacteriologic diseases, including tuberculosis. In the 1950s, Americans celebrated Jonas Salk's team when they announced a vaccine for polio, a disabling and deadly disease that paralyzed and killed children and young adults.[10] Millions of children lined up to receive their shots, becoming polio pioneers.

These rapid changes during the first half of the twentieth century resulted in environmental therapeutics fading from popular view and medical practice. The beach, with its restorative sea breezes and invigorating saltwater, seemed to hearken to a time before magic bullet drugs. The shift in thinking was so profound that by 1939 journalists were announcing, as if for the first time, that a physician could, and perhaps should, prescribe vacation sites.

In June 1939, the *Science News-Letter*, a popular science magazine, published an article entitled "Prescribed Vacations." Reporter Jane Stafford stoked her readers' curiosity, writing, "Rx: 10 days at the shore—to be taken as directed." She goaded her readers to continue, tantalizing them with a suggestion: "Here's a new idea for that summer vacation you are planning: Have it made to order for you according to your doctor's prescription."[11] Stafford then summarized a recent article from the *Journal of the American Medical Association* in which physician Charles I. Singer advocated for Americans to consult a doctor before selecting a vacation destination.

Stafford framed a medical prescription for travel as a new idea. The public ostensibly needed to be taught to seek a physician's advice before traveling.[12] Yet not even twenty years earlier urban children and mothers had sought such prescriptions to seaside hospitals. According to Singer, the medical profession needed to be reminded as well. In March 1939, the *Journal of the American Medical Association* published Singer's article "Medically Supervised Vacational Migrations." Singer opened his article by imploring his colleagues take advantage of vacations' popularity, noting that more than 35 million Americans spent more than $5 billion on vacations. He defined travel as a prime medical tool that could improve chronically ill patients' health and bolster the fitness of healthy individuals. Singer wrote that depending on where patients resided, travel could be invigorating or sedative and result in changes to patients' metabolism. Singer's claims followed a pattern similar to those of marine medication practitioners from earlier decades; so too does his list of patients who benefited from a sedative climate. He noted that "the feeble aged and . . . the delicate child," as well as patients with rheumatic heart disease, chronic nephritis, and rheumatoid arthritis, all improved by moving to a relaxing environment.[13]

Singer either dismissed or was simply unaware of the vast literature on practices like marine medication. He lamented that "these migrations are not studied from a medical point of view." However, he echoed concerns of predecessors, including surgeon John Packard, who bemoaned when vacationers did not seek direction or medical supervision. Singer further acknowledged that Americans traveled primarily for "wanderlust and the craving for a good time." Singer outlined a plan for training practitioners in climatology, the types of institutions that would serve vacationers, and how prescribing vacations could benefit the public, medical science, the medical profession, and health resorts.[14]

Singer's medical colleagues seemed to pay little attention to the article, despite the American Medical Association actually having a committee on spas and health resorts.[15] The article provides hints as to why his recommendations failed to gain traction in the United States. According to Singer, the United States lacked coordinated efforts that supported travel prescriptions. This wasn't simply the result of scientific advances, as European physicians and governments simultaneously maintained their support of scientific studies of climate and environmental health institutions. Singer enumerated Europe's numerous commitments, which included collaboration between personal physicians and practitioners at spas and health resorts; European spas' provision of mandatory medical exams, supervision, and case histories; German universities' climate research stations; a coordination of public services in France to provide sick children access to thousands of beds in spas and health resorts; Hungary's health insurance for the chronically ill; and Austria's national committee on mineral springs and muds. Singer also stated that Belgium alone supported "forty seashore sanatoriums for underdeveloped, sickly children on the 40 miles of seashore."[16] The United States, in contrast, boasted no such nationally coordinated efforts.

Stafford's and Singer's articles suggests how much popular and medical perceptions had changed in the United States in just half a century. There are likely many nuances left to uncover during the span of the twentieth century that fall beyond the scope of this book. We know that forms of environmental therapeutics still existed beyond 1940. Before the public had access to antibiotics, sanitariums continued to care for tuberculous patients in the mountains and at the seashore. Likewise, springs and spas catered to patients who suffered from chronic conditions, and Americans with tuberculosis, asthma, and hay fever sought relief in the desert or mountains.[17]

Equally telling, seashore and floating hospitals continued to operate in the northeastern corridor of the United States. The Children's Seashore House remained on the beach at Atlantic City until 1990, when it closed its seaside location and transferred operations to Philadelphia when it merged with the Children's Hospital of Philadelphia. The New York Floating Hospital remained on a ship in New York's harbor until September 11, 2001, when it could not secure a safe place to dock in the wake of the terrorist attacks on the World Trade Center towers. The Boston Floating Hospital arrived in the city after a fire destroyed its ship in the 1920s. It cared for Boston's children until 2022, when it closed its inpatient beds.[18]

The relocation of seashore hospitals into cities is emblematic. Americans maintained some of these medical institutions, even if they lost sight of the environmental ideologies that structured their foundations. In urban hospitals, UV lamps dot the walls, and bags of saline hang from shiny metal poles. Twenty-first-century Americans are surrounded by vestiges of environmental therapeutics and medical ideologies, but we have obscured their place-based origins.

It is also difficult to scientifically study the holistic impact of environments on health and well-being. Increasingly, however, people are trying. Nearly simultaneous with Donaldson's discovery, journalist Richard Louv published his book *Last Child in the Woods: Saving Our Children from Nature-Deficit Disorder*. "Nature deficit disorder" is not a medical diagnosis but a turn of phrase that Louv coined to capture an emerging scientific and medical sentiment. Louv collated studies about the health benefits of outdoor play and concluded that children's health improves after spending time playing outside, in unstructured environments.[19]

Last Child in the Woods became a national best seller, won the Audubon Medal for "sounding the alarm" about the medical costs of keeping children away from the natural world, and inspired a television series.[20] These successes suggest that the book tapped into existing sentiments. Reviewers reported that Louv provided them with scientific evidence of what they had long suspected. One person wrote, "A great read—maybe because it matches so much with my view that for a full and complete life we need to learn how to connect with the natural world we live in."[21] Another reader, Joyce, summarized that "Louv gives a name (nature-deficit disorder) to the staggering divide that has developed between children and the outdoors and links the absence of nature in the lives of today's children to the disturbing childhood trends of obesity, attention disorders, and depression." She concludes her review with a line of deep technological pessimism, writing, "I say we shall rue the day we moved indoors and in front of screens."[22]

Newspaper articles picked up these threads about the health benefits of natural outdoor environments. In 2015, the *New York Times* published an article by Gretchen Reynolds titled "How Walking in Nature Changes the Brain." She reported that scientists determined that "a walk in the park may soothe the mind and, in the process, change the workings of our brains in ways that improve our mental health." Reynolds explained that people living in cities who spent little time in "green, natural spaces" had "higher risk for anxiety, depression and other mental illnesses," as compared to people who reside in nonurban environments.[23]

Reynolds referenced a study led by Gregory Bratman, then a graduate student at Stanford University. Bratman concluded that people who walked in a "lush, green portion of the Stanford campus were more attentive and happier afterward than volunteers who strolled for the same amount of time near heavy traffic."[24] Bratman's study was well received. In addition to Reynolds's *New York Times* article, scholars have cited the study more than a thousand times since in 2015.[25] Howard Frumkin, a physician, public health expert, and environmental health advocate, used the study as the basis for "a research agenda on nature contact and health, identifying principal domains of research and key questions that, if answered, would provide the basis for evidence-based public health interventions."[26]

Other physicians were also working on how to connect patients with healthy outdoor settings. In the 2010s, a group of California physicians built on the idea that time outside benefited patients. They founded ParkRx to help support practitioners identify local programs and places that linked patients with parks and outdoor programs. By the end of the decade there were park prescription programs across the United States, and the group maintained a website to facilitate the identification of green spaces.[27]

Ironically, the global COVID-19 pandemic that began in 2020 may have halted that trajectory. During the pandemic, Americans rediscovered that being outdoors was not only safer but healthier. They did what others had done for centuries. Urbanites who could afford to abandon the city left for homes in less populous places. As administrators and school boards scrambled to open schools, some built outdoor classrooms capitalizing on fresh air and lower rates of contagion; people expressed surprise upon discovering there was historical precedent for the plan.[28] Additionally, once people began to travel, many sought refuge in nature. Visitors swarmed America's national parks and crowded its shorelines. Despite a surging interest in spending time outdoors, support for park prescription programs faltered, suggesting that the US medical system lacked an infrastructure to facilitate or maintain its success.

Despite the struggle to prescribe nature, medical geographers, public health experts, and physicians are increasingly studying the impact of our environment and climate change on health. They are tracing the potential benefits of green and blue spaces. Their findings are inspiring some doctors to reexamine centuries-old practices like *shinrin-yoku*, the Japanese practice of "forest bathing," to determine its therapeutic potential.[29] Meanwhile, medical geographers are analyzing the health benefits of naturally occurring blue spaces, including oceans, lakes, and rivers.[30]

Building on the consensus that exposure to outdoor elements could improve health, in 2024 *The Atlantic* reported that public health officials in Australia and Europe were once again encouraging people to sunbathe. Scientists discovered that natural sun exposure results in lower rates of multiple sclerosis and other autoimmune diseases. This is a stark reversal from decades-long campaigns. Across the global West, medical and public health officials have long advised people to avoid sun exposure and to cover oneself in sunscreen and protective clothing because of potentially cancerous UV rays.[31] These contradictory recommendations reflect a twenty-first-century quagmire of risk-benefit calculations. Which is worse? Potentially developing skin cancer or multiple sclerosis? While scientists have aggregated data about how MS risk goes up the higher the latitude of one's residence, population data may not apply to any one individual.

We know that bodies respond differently to the same external stimuli. Studying why this happens may yield fruitful data, but quantitatively precise measures often fail to capture the holistic set of interactions that occur between people's bodies and their environments. A 2017 article in *Environmental Research* acknowledges this tension. The public health experts who authored the paper concluded that green space is beneficial to health but that "much remains to be learned about the specific pathways and functional form of such relationships, and how these may vary by context, population groups and health outcomes."[32]

As environmental historians have noted, bodies, like environments, are messy. The effect of the seashore and outdoor play on the multivariable elements of health are difficult to represent in clinical language.[33] Neither the environment nor the human body follows predictable—much less standardized—pathways in response to exposures. By relying on "specific pathways and functional form," we risk not being able to appreciate the impact of the whole environment on our bodies and health.[34]

Quantifiable data has value, and basing programs on evidence is good policy. However, relying solely on numerical outcomes narrows our vision. Looking back can offer us a way forward.[35] History teaches us that there are other bodies of evidence that have historically counted.[36] As we have learned, parents and families have sought health not only in complex treatment regimens and sterilized hospital rooms but also in the bracing ocean air of America's northeastern seashore. Today's medical proof will not be ruddy cheeks and rounded bellies, but we could imagine systems in which perceptions and experience constitute evidence, where qualitative, experiential data complements quantitative metrics. We could count patients' embodied knowledge. We can learn from people like Mallory Smith, who embraced the seashore to enhance her health. Living with cystic fibrosis, Smith reflected that the "ocean has been my escape, my passion, and a powerful healing agent."[37] Physicians could, like Donaldson, acknowledge that their experiments derived from an awareness of environmentally derived benefits. We can decide to put the environment back into the medical equation.

As we confront the realities of climate change, the history of America's northeastern seashore reminds us that there are other ways to value, know, and appreciate our environments. At the beach, we are immersed in the sunlight, sea air, and at times the seawater, not just UV rays, ozone, and saline. We bathe in breezes, experience the shock of cold water, and feel the pleasure and relaxation of time outside, in the sand and under the sun. The same holds true for forests, mountaintops, and even cities. While we may not be able to pinpoint the precise mechanisms by which blue and green spaces promote health and well-being (or the ways that cities might deplete it), we can also use our common sense and experiences to guide us toward a new way of knowing landscapes through our physical and psychological responses. If we do, we might regain a shared understanding that places like the beach can cure us, if we care for them.

NOTES

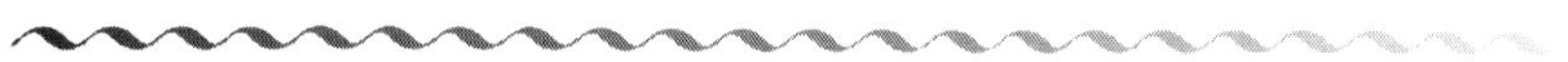

Introduction

1. "7-Year-Old Girl Dies after Getting Trapped in Sand at Lauderdale-by-the-Sea Beach," NBC6 (South Florida), February 20, 2024, https://www.nbcmiami.com/news/local/kids-trapped-sand-lauderdale-by-the-sea-beach/3238718.

2. Corbin, *Lure of the Sea*.

3. Aron, *Working at Play*, 20–21.

4. Kasson, *Amusing the Million*.

5. Ritchie, *Lure of the Beach*, 2–4.

6. Brochard, *Sea-Air and Sea-Bathing for Children and Invalids*.

7. Seashore hospitals were popular in the United States, Europe, and Argentina. See Crnic and Connolly, "'They Can't Help Getting Well Here'"; Nelson and Förhammar, "Swedish Seaside Sanatoria"; Reber, "Poor, Ill, and Sometimes Abandoned"; Vanobbergen, "Belgian Sea Hospitals"; and Vanobbergen and Vansieleghem, "Repairing the Body."

8. Parascandola and Crnic, "Coney Island Babies."

9. Ritchie, *Lure of the Beach*, chap. 3.

10. Kiechle, *Smell Detectives*, esp. chap. 7.

11. Rosenberg, *Cholera Years*; Leavitt, *Typhoid Mary*; Willoughby, *Yellow Fever, Race, and Ecology*.

12. Melosi, *Sanitary City*; Tarr, *Search for the Ultimate Sink*; Leavitt, *Healthiest City*.

13. Greene, *Horses at Work*; McNeur, *Taming Manhattan*.

14. Kiechle, "Navigating by Nose."

15. Kiechle, *Smell Detectives*.

16. Bernstein, "Health Activism from the Bottom Up," 317–44.

17. Bean, "Walter Reed and the Ordeal of Human Experiments"; Hammonds, *Childhood's Deadly Scourge*.

18. Tomes, *Gospel of Germs*; Worboys, *Spreading Germs*.

19. Here I am inspired by Aaron Antonovsky's critique of a more contemporary medical focus on disease causation and the "pathogenic," rather than "salutogenic," approach to health. See Antonovsky, "Salutogenic Model as a Theory."

20. This book builds on and contributes to scholarship on the history of environments and health. In particular see Valenčius, *Health of the Country*; Mitman, *Breathing Space*; Nash, *Inescapable Ecologies*; Sellers, "To Place or Not to Place"; and Sellers, "Thoreau's Body."

21. Mitman, "Hay Fever Holiday."

22. Cronon, "Trouble with Wilderness."

23. This idea builds on the urban-rural dichotomy, which has a deep history that has attracted considerable analysis; see Cronon, *Nature's Metropolis*; R. Williams, *Country and the City*; and Lears, *Rebirth of a Nation*.

24. Sears, *Sacred Places*.

25. Benson, *Surroundings*.

26. Kasson, *Amusing the Million*; Simon, *Boardwalk of Dreams*.

27. An intriguing question would be the similarities and differences in health practices, contrasting beliefs, and practices surrounding fresh versus salt water. See Wright, *SickKids*.

28. Simon, *Boardwalk of Dreams*; Aron, *Working at Play*; Mitman, "Hay Fever Holiday"; Shaffer, *See America First*; Valenčius, "Gender and the Economy of Health."

29. Peiss, *Cheap Amusements*; Schlichting, *New York Recentered*; Fisher, *Urban Green*.

30. Duane, *Children's Table*.

ONE *Cities and the Pathology of Place*

1. *Thirty-Eighth Annual Report of the Managers of the Sanitarium Association of Philadelphia* (Philadelphia: Allen, Lane and Scott, 1913), 10–12. (Other such reports hereafter cited as *Annual Report of the SAP*, with the appropriate year and page number.)

2. *Annual Report of the SAP*, 1902, 11.

3. *Annual Report of the SAP*, 1913, 10–12. The quotes are consolidated but taken from the annual report. Other details, such as the distance to the sanitarium and popularity of the association, have been supplemented by other years' annual reports.

4. Riney-Kehrberg, *Nature of Childhood*, 58.

5. Nasaw, *Children of the City*.

6. Dyl, "War on Rats versus the Right to Keep Chickens"; B. Hansen, "America's First Medical Breakthrough."

7. Kiechle, *Smell Detectives*.

8. Benson, *Surroundings*, chap. 3. For an overview of the history of social work, see Abrams and Curran, "Between Women"; and Ehrenreich, *Altruistic Imagination*.

9. Riney-Kehrberg, *Nature of Childhood*.

10. R. Williams, *Country and the City*; Cronon, *Nature's Metropolis*; Schlichting, *New York Recentered*.

11. Spirn, "Constructing Nature."

12. Zelizer, *Pricing the Priceless Child.*

13. Dye and Smith, "Mother Love and Infant Death."

14. Brosco, "Sin or Folly," 76; Decennial Census Historical Facts, 1930, US Bureau of the Census, https://www.census.gov/history/www/through_the_decades/fast_facts/1930_fast_facts.html.

15. For the interactions of public health, immigration, and the Immigration Act of 1924, see Fairchild, "Policies of Inclusion."

16. For more on this time period in general, see Hofstadter, *Age of Reform*; Hays, *Conservation and the Gospel of Efficiency*; and Boyer, *Urban Masses and Moral Order in America.*

17. Porter, *Greatest Benefit to Mankind*, 122–24, 234–35.

18. Minardi, "Boston Inoculation Controversy of 1721–1722."

19. Pernick, "Politics, Parties, and Pestilence"; Willoughby, *Yellow Fever, Race, and Ecology.*

20. For examples of epidemics and their impact, see Rogers, *Dirt and Disease*; and Rosenberg, *Cholera Years.*

21. Dye and Smith, "Mother Love and Infant Death"; Meckel, *Save the Babies.*

22. Condran and Murphy, "Defining and Managing Infant Mortality," 477.

23. Mortality Statistics, 1900 to 1904, Bureau of the Census, US Department of Commerce and Labor, 1906, in "Achievements in Public Health, 1900–1999: Control of Infectious Diseases," *MMWR Weekly* 48, no. 29 (1999), https://www.cdc.gov/mmwr/preview/mmwrhtml/mm4829a1.htm; "America's Health Rankings," annual report of the United Health Foundation, 2018, https://www.americashealthrankings.org/learn/reports/2018-annual-report/findings-international-comparison; "Infant Mortality," Centers for Disease Control, accessed October 28, 2024, https://www.cdc.gov/maternal-infant-health/infant-mortality/?CDC_AAref_Val=https://www.cdc.gov/reproductivehealth/maternalinfanthealth/infantmortality.htm.

24. Condran and Murphy, "Defining and Managing Infant Mortality," 483–87.

25. Rosenberg, "Tyranny of Diagnosis."

26. Warren, *Starved for Light*, chap. 1, which is titled "Coeval with Civilization: Rickets from Ancient Egypt to the 'Dark Satanic Mills.'"

27. Palm, "Geographical Distributions and Etiology of Rickets," 271. While Palm acknowledged that rickets was generally considered "rare" in the United States, he asserted that "the malady is met with as commonly in Philadelphia as in the large towns of Europe" (273).

28. Palm, "Geographical Distributions and Etiology of Rickets," 335.

29. Semba, "Impact of Improved Nutrition on Disease Prevention," 164–65.

30. Semba, "Impact of Improved Nutrition on Disease Prevention," 164.

31. See the papers in the multivolume *Transactions of the Sixth International Congress on Tuberculosis.*

32. Robison, "Ocean Climates," 1244–45.

33. Nissenbaum, *Sex, Diet, and Debility in Jacksonian America*, 54–57; LaFay, "Afflictions of the Tropics' Brink," esp. chaps. 3 and 4.

34. American practitioners did not view this as a disease of childhood, but Dutch doctors did diagnose children with the condition; see Bakker, "Before Ritalin"; and Schuster, *Neurasthenic Nation*.

35. Mintz, *Huck's Raft*; Brooks-Gunn and Duncan Johnson, "G. Stanley Hall's Contribution to Science, Practice, and Policy."

36. Markowitz and Rosner, *Lead Wars*. In a more recent related matter, a panic regarding gas stoves dominated media in the early months of 2023; see Maxine Joselow, with Vanessa Montalbano, "Gas Stove Pollution Causes 12.7% of Childhood Asthma, Study Finds," *Washington Post*, January 6, 2023, https://www.washingtonpost.com/politics/2023/01/06/gas-stove-pollution-causes-127-childhood-asthma-study-finds/.

37. S. Baker, "Importance of Good Health," 35. On ideas of the plasticity of children, see Crnic, "Better Babies."

38. Melosi, *Sanitary City*, 71–128.

39. Carr, *Topography of Wellness*, 11–31.

40. Jain, "Dangerous Instrumentality."

41. Zelizer, *Pricing the Priceless Child*, 35.

42. Zelizer, *Pricing the Priceless Child*, 47–48.

43. Schweik, *Ugly Laws*. There is ample room in the field for scholars who are interested in interrogating the intersection of environment, health, and disability. Some literature on which to build includes Linker, "On the Borderland of Medical and Disability History"; Borsay and Dale, *Disabled Children*; Koven, "Remembering and Dismemberment"; and Byrom, "Progressive Movement and the Child with Physical Disabilities."

44. Kelley, "Street Trader under Illinois Law," 297–98.

45. Nasaw, *Children of the City*.

46. Brooks-Gunn and Duncan Johnson, "G. Stanley Hall's Contributions to Science, Practice, and Policy," 247.

47. Zinguer, "The Sandbox."

48. Spencer-Wood, "Turn of the Century Women's Organizations," 130.

49. Zinguer, "The Sandbox," 28.

50. Zinguer, "The Sandbox"; Spencer-Wood, "Turn of the Century Women's Organizations," 130.

51. Gutman, *City for Children*, 217–18.

52. Flanagan, "City Profitable."

53. Hall, *Story of a Sand-pile*, 3.

54. Zueblin, "City Child at Play," 447.

55. Nasaw, *Children of the City*.

56. Zueblin, "City Child at Play," 443.

57. Zueblin, "City Child at Play," 448. His framing of his claims in terms of poten-

tials also brushes against eugenic thinking that was prominent at the time. Lombardo, *Three Generations, No Imbeciles*; D. Kevles, *In the Name of Eugenics*. In the context of children, see Stern, "Making Better Babies."

58. Zueblin, "City Child at Play," 443. On children's interaction with urban spaces, see Riney-Kehrberg, *Nature of Childhood*. Urban parks have received more general attention; see Cranz, *Politics of Park Design*; and Spirn, *Granite Garden*.

59. Spirn, "Constructing Nature."

60. Zueblin, "City Child at Play," 444.

61. Zueblin, "City Child at Play," 444.

62. Zueblin, "City Child at Play," 447.

63. Cavallo, *Muscles and Morals*; Carr, *Topography of Wellness*, 43–53.

64. Atkins, *Out of the Cradle into the World*, 24.

65. Atkins, *Out of the Cradle into the World*, 74.

66. Atkins, *Out of the Cradle into the World*, 79.

67. Atkins, *Out of the Cradle into the World*, 76.

68. Atkins, *Out of the Cradle into the World*, 76.

69. Nasaw, *Children of the City*.

70. Riney-Kehrberg, *Nature of Childhood*, 47.

71. Kelley, "Street Trader under Illinois Law," 295.

72. Stradling, *Smokestacks and Progressives*, 5.

73. Waldo Frank, *Our America* (New York: Boni & Liveright, 1919) and Frangipani Soot [pseud.], letter to the editor, *Milwaukee Sentinel*, October 28, 1888, both quoted in Stradling, *Smokestacks and Progressives*, 22.

74. Madrigal, "Aghast over Beijing's Air Pollution?"

75. Adams, *Architecture in the Family Way*.

76. Kiechle, *Smell Detectives*, esp. chap. 3; Hoy, *Chasing Dirt*.

77. Cowan, *More Work for Mother*.

78. Adams, *Architecture in the Family Way*; Ogle, *All the Modern Conveniences*.

79. Social Service Reports, Women's Auxiliary of the Hospital of the University of Pennsylvania, Ward G, December 1921, 1, Barbara Bates Center for the Study of the History of Nursing, School of Nursing, University of Pennsylvania, Philadelphia (cited hereafter as HUP Ward G, plus date and page information).

80. HUP Ward G, December 1921, 1.

81. HUP Ward G, December 1921, 1–2.

82. HUP Ward G, January 1919, 1. After at first writing the name "Lucy," the report's author switches to calling the girl "Lizzie." I use "Lucy" since that is how it first appears in the record. Infant feeding was one of the many topics of maternal education at the time. See, for instance, Apple, *Mothers and Medicine*.

83. Katz, *In the Shadow of the Poorhouse*; Boyer, *Urban Masses and Moral Order in America*; Kraut, *Silent Travelers*.

84. HUP Ward G, April 1921, 2.

85. Mothers have often been blamed; see Ladd-Taylor and Umansky, *"Bad" Mothers.*

86. HUP Ward G, March 1922.

87. Other scholars, including Mitman, "Hay Fever Holiday," have noted this phenomenon.

88. Stradling, *Making Mountains*; Peña, "Recharging at the Fordyce."

89. Plater, "Tonic for Body or Soul," 1.

90. Guarneri, "Changing Strategies for Child Welfare"; Shearer, *Two Weeks Every Summer*; on leisure corridors, see Schlichting, *New York Recentered.*

91. R. Fulton Cutting, "From Stifling Tenement to Seashore and Country," n.d., in author's personal collection.

92. Cutting, "From Stifling Tenement to Seashore and Country."

93. *Annual Report of the SAP*, 1883, 6.

94. *Annual Report of the SAP*, 1884, 34–35.

95. *Annual Report of the SAP*, 1886, 10.

96. *Annual Report of the SAP*, 1888, 6.

97. *Annual Report of the SAP*, 1883, 24–25.

98. *Annual Report of the SAP*, 1883, 26–27.

99. *Annual Report of the SAP*, 1883, 16.

100. *Annual Report of the SAP*, 1883, 16.

101. *Annual Report of the SAP*, 1883, 17.

102. M. Plater makes this argument with regard to the Boston Floating Hospital. They also present a compelling analysis of how the Fresh Air Fund used "fresh air" more symbolically than medically; see Plater, "Tonic for Body or Soul," 865–90.

103. *A Brief History of the Boston Floating Hospital* (pamphlet), 1906, 5, available online at the National Library of Medicine, http://resource.nlm.nih.gov/101725502.

104. Theiss, "Least of These," 546.

105. Theiss, "Least of These," 545.

106. Quoted in Theiss, "Least of These," 543.

107. Quoted in Theiss, "Least of These," 542.

108. Sara Jensen Carr also makes this point in her 2021 book *The Topography of Wellness.*

109. Massachusetts Emergency and Hygiene Association, *Fifth Annual Report*, 1889, 31, as quoted in Zinguer, "The Sandbox," 29.

TWO *Finding Cures at the Shore*

1. Corbin, *Lure of the Sea*, 2.

2. Corbin, *Lure of the Sea*, 85–94.

3. Corbin, *Lure of the Sea*, 61–62.

4. Aron, *Working at Play*, 21–22.

5. Mitman, "Hay Fever Holiday"; Valenčius, "Gender and the Economy of Health."

6. Donegan, *Hydropathic Highway to Health*; Peña, "Recharging at the Fordyce"; Porter, "Medical History of Waters and Spas"; Weisz, "Spas, Mineral Waters, and Hydrological Science"; Herbert, "Gender and the Spa."

7. Rothman, *Living in the Shadow of Death*, chap. 2.

8. Brochard, *Sea-Air and Sea-Bathing for Children and Invalids.*

9. This type of scientific effort fit within the general trend of reductionism at this time; see Lawrence and Weisz, *Greater than the Parts.*

10. Hinsdale, *Atmospheric Air in Relation to Tuberculosis*, 48–49.

11. Sloane, "'Not Designed Merely to Heal.'"

12. On the history of children's health and pediatrics, see Halpern, *American Pediatrics*; Stern and Markel, *Formative Years*; Golden, Meckel, and Prescott, *Children and Youth in Sickness and in Health.*

13. For a contemporary perspective on rabies, see "Clinical Overview of Rabies," Centers for Disease Control, accessed October 29, 2024, https://www.cdc.gov/rabies/symptoms/index.html.

14. B. Hansen, "America's First Medical Breakthrough," 384.

15. Only four of the children were determined to need Pasteur's treatment. B. Hansen, "America's First Medical Breakthrough," 389.

16. "The Dog-Bitten Children: How M. Pasteur Inoculated the Four Patients in Their Stomachs," *Macon Telegraph*, December 25, 1885.

17. "Pasteur's Patients: Return Home of the Four Newark Boys," *Philadelphia Inquirer*, January 15, 1886.

18. On incubators, see J. Baker, *Machine in the Nursery*; and Golden, *Babies Made Us Modern.*

19. "A Cheerful View of a Serious Situation," *Gunter's Magazine Advertiser*, vol. 8, 1906.

20. Koch was, and remains, widely credited for the discovery of the cholera bacillus, although some recent articles have sought to restore credit to Italian physician Filippo Pacini as the first to isolate and identify the bacterium during an 1854 cholera outbreak. Carboni, "Enigma of Pacini's *Vibrio cholerae* Discovery."

21. Bornside, "Jaime Ferran and Preventive Inoculation against Cholera."

22. Feudtner, *Bittersweet.*

23. Rosenberg, *Care of Strangers*; Brandt and Sloane, "Of Beds and Benches"; Sloane, "'Not Designed Merely to Heal.'" On hospitals in the twentieth century, see Stevens, *In Sickness and in Wealth.*

24. Howell, *Technology in the Hospital.*

25. Tomes, *Gospel of Germs.*

26. *Annual Report for the Year 1875: The Children's Sea Shore House at Atlantic City*, 13 (cited hereafter as *CSH Annual Report*, plus the relevant year and page number, and available at the Historical Society of Pennsylvania Archives, Philadelphia); Brochard, *Sea-Air and Sea-Bathing for Children and Invalids.*

27. Brochard, *Sea-Air and Sea-Bathing for Children and Invalids*, 103–28. For an

example of a book published for a general audience on marine medication, see Packard, *Sea Air and Sea Bathing*. This book was published as part of a series, American Health Primers, meant to teach a general audience about how to properly practice preventive health measures.

28. Oliver, "Therapeutics of the Sea-Side."

29. William Bennett, the physician in charge of the Children's Seashore House, trained at the top institutions in the United States, furthered his education in Europe, and became one of the earliest US specialists in pediatrics. D. Miller, "Memoir of Dr. William Henry Bennett."

30. "History of the Children's Seashore House," in *CSH Annual Report*, 1918.

31. For more on this, see LaFay, "Afflictions of the Tropics' Brink," chap. 2; and Livingston, *Debility and the Moral Imagination in Botswana*. In the context of Victorian cities, see Rosen, "Disease, Debility, and Death."

32. Oliver, "Therapeutics of the Sea-Side," 551.

33. Robison, "Ocean Climates," 1245.

34. *CSH Annual Report*, 1882, 13.

35. Oliver, "Therapeutics of the Sea-Side," 551.

36. Oliver, "Therapeutics of the Sea-Side," 550–51.

37. *CSH Annual Report*, 1887, 6.

38. *CSH Annual Report*, 1887, 6; *CSH Annual Report*, 1910, 17–19.

39. *CSH Annual Report*, 1887, 5–6.

40. *CSH Annual Report*, 1910, 17.

41. *CSH Annual Report*, 1910, 18–19.

42. See, e.g., Reed, "Diseased Conditions for Which Sea Air Is of Doubtful Benefit."

43. The literature on tuberculosis is vast. See, e.g., Ott, *Fevered Lives*; Bates, *Bargaining for Life*; and Rothman, *Living in the Shadow of Death*. On children and tuberculosis, see Connolly, *Saving Sickly Children*.

44. Oliver, "Therapeutics of the Sea-Side," 551.

45. Reed, "Effects of Sea Air upon Diseases of the Respiratory Organs," 57. Philadelphia physician W. Blair Stewart agreed with Boardman. In 1900 Stewart argued that patients in the early stages of pulmonary tuberculosis improved with sea-air and sun exposure at Atlantic City and concurred that the marine environment was detrimental for patients with advanced stages of the disease.

46. *CSH Annual Report*, 1910, 9.

47. *CSH Annual Report*, 1882, 14. People were concerned in general about disabled bodies during this time, as documented in Linker, *War's Waste*, 38–51; and Koven, "Remembering and Dismemberment."

48. Shands, "DeForest Willard, Philadelphia's Pioneer Orthopaedic Surgeon."

49. *CSH Annual Report*, 1895, 10.

50. *CSH Annual Report*, 1911, 15.

51. Brosco, "Weight Charts and Well-Child Care"; Weaver, "In the Balance."

52. Reed, "Effects of Sea Air upon Diseases of the Respiratory Organs," 54.

53. *CSH Annual Report*, 1915, app.; Brannan, "Seashore and Fresh Air Treatment."

54. *CSH Annual Report*, 1883, 11–12.

55. *CSH Annual Report*, 1917, 19.

56. Hammond, "Seashore Treatment of Osteomyelitis."

57. A. Miller, "Seashore Treatment of the Tubercular Arthritis of Children," 659.

58. For a general background on orthopedics, see Cooter, *Surgery and Society in Peace and War*.

59. A. Miller, "Seashore Treatment of the Tubercular Arthritis of Children," 659.

60. A. Miller, "Seashore Treatment of the Tubercular Arthritis of Children," 660.

61. A. Miller, "Seashore Treatment of the Tubercular Arthritis of Children," 660.

62. A. Miller, "Seashore Treatment of the Tubercular Arthritis of Children," 661.

63. Whitbeck, "Review of the Ten Years' Work at Sea Breeze Hospital."

64. Whitbeck, "Review of the Ten Years' Work at Sea Breeze Hospital," 124.

65. Whitbeck, "Review of the Ten Years' Work at Sea Breeze Hospital," 124.

66. Hammond, "Treatment of Bone Tuberculosis at the Crawford Allen Hospital," 50.

67. Vogel and Rosenberg, *Therapeutic Revolution*; Warner, *Therapeutic Perspective*.

68. Stewart, "Influence of Sea-Air and Sea-Water Baths on Disease," 678–79.

69. Brochard, *Sea-Air and Sea-Bathing for Children and Invalids*, 83.

70. Increasing attention has recently been given to cold-water bathing or so-called polar plunges. Advocates report both mental and physical benefits. These articles also highlight our contemporary skepticism that such environmental experiences may be therapeutic. See, for instance, Chloe Williams, "Cold Water Plunges Are Trendy: Can They Really Reduce Anxiety and Depression?," *New York Times*, February 20, 2022.

71. Brochard, *Sea-Air and Sea-Bathing for Children and Invalids*, 83.

72. Brochard, *Sea-Air and Sea-Bathing for Children and Invalids*, 83; Stewart, "Influence of Sea-Air and Sea-Water Baths on Disease," 679.

73. Stewart, "Influence of Sea-Air and Sea-Water Baths on Disease," 679.

74. *CSH Annual Report*, 1875, 15.

75. Brochard, *Sea-Air and Sea-Bathing for Children and Invalids*, 86–87.

76. Packard, *Sea-Air and Sea-Bathing*.

77. Gauvain, "Sea Bathing in the Treatment of Surgical Tuberculosis."

78. Gauvain, "Hastings Popular Lecture on Sun, Air, and Sea Bathing," 60.

79. Gauvain, "Hastings Popular Lecture on Sun, Air, and Sea Bathing," 60–61.

80. Hill and Campbell with Gauvain, "Metabolism of Children Undergoing Open-Air Treatment."

81. Hill and Campbell with Gauvain, "Metabolism of Children Undergoing Open-Air Treatment," 303. On acclimatization, see Gauvain, "Hastings Popular Lecture on Sun, Air, and Sea Bathing," 60.

82. Hill and Campbell with Gauvain, "Metabolism of Children Undergoing Open-Air Treatment," 303.

83. Guarneri, "Changing Strategies for Child Welfare."
84. Reed, "Effects of Sea Air upon Diseases of the Respiratory Organs," 51.
85. Kiechle, "'Nature's Great Disinfectant'"; Thorsheim, *Inventing Pollution*, 22–25.
86. Reed, "Effects of Sea Air upon Diseases of the Respiratory Organs," 54.
87. Several authors discuss this blending; see, e.g., Tomes, *Gospel of Germs*.
88. Reed, "Effects of Sea Air upon Diseases of the Respiratory Organs," 51.
89. Reed, "Effects of Sea Air upon Diseases of the Respiratory Organs."
90. Stewart, "Influence of Sea-Air and Sea-Water Baths on Disease," 678.
91. Rollier, *Heliotherapy*, 22–24.
92. Downes and Blunt, "Researches on the Effect of Light upon Bacteria and Other Organisms," 496–97.
93. Woloshyn, "Patients Rebuilt"; Freund, *American Sunshine*.
94. Hammond, "Heliotherapy (of Rollier) as an Adjunct in the Treatment of Bone Disease," 272.
95. Hammond, "Heliotherapy (of Rollier) as an Adjunct in the Treatment of Bone Disease," 272.
96. Gauvain, "Sea Bathing in the Treatment of Surgical Tuberculosis," 60.
97. Gauvain, "Sea Bathing in the Treatment of Surgical Tuberculosis," 60; Richards, *Euthenics, the Science of Controllable Environment*; Munns, "'Not by a Decree of Fate'"; Weigley, "It Might Have Been Euthenics."
98. A. Miller, "Seashore Treatment of the Tubercular Arthritis of Children," 659.
99. *CSH Annual Report*, 1912, 16.
100. Sellers, "To Place or Not to Place."

THREE *The Shifting Sands of Health Tourism*

1. *Atlantic City and County, New Jersey, Biographically Illustrated.*
2. Simon, *Boardwalk of Dreams*.
3. Simon, "Natural History of the Life and Death of a Great American City."
4. Simon, "Natural History of the Life and Death of a Great American City."
5. *CSH Annual Report*, 1898, 27.
6. Grover, *Hard at Play*.
7. Simon, *Boardwalk of Dreams*, 22.
8. Some historians take the claims more seriously than others but even then do not engage with health as a central point of analysis. See Aron, *Working at Play*; Funnell, *By the Beautiful Sea*; Shaffer, *See America First*; and Stradling, *Making Mountains*.
9. Scholars who are interested in health seeking are an important and notable counterpoint within the history of tourism; see Valenčius, "Gender and the Economy on the Santa Fe Trail"; and Mitman, "Hay Fever Holiday."
10. Funnell, *By the Beautiful Sea*, 4; Winpenny, "Engineer as Promoter."
11. *Atlantic City and County, New Jersey, Biographically Illustrated*, 44.

12. Jones, "'Lungs of the City'"; Keichle, *Smell Detectives*, 30–33.

13. Funnell, *By the Beautiful Sea*, 3–6.

14. Sears, *Sacred Places*.

15. Ethan Carr, "Olmsted and Scenic Preservation," WNED, Buffalo-Toronto Public Media, 2014, https://www.wned.org/television/wned-productions/wned-history-productions/frederick-law-olmsted-designing-america/learn-more-olmsted/olmsted-and-scenic-preservation/.

16. Muir, *The Yosemite*, 256.

17. Lewis, "Beach at Atlantic City," 764.

18. Snodgrass, *Civil War Era and Reconstruction*, 302. In 1865, the readership of *Harper's Weekly* was three hundred thousand.

19. Philadelphia Railroad, *Atlantic City, N.J.: The Great American Sea-Side Resort* (Philadelphia: Press of Allen, Lane, and Scott, 1894), accessed at https://hdl.handle.net/2027/njp.32101072334038.

20. Funnell, *By the Beautiful Sea*, 135–37; Simon, *Boardwalk of Dreams*, 22–24; Aron, *Working at Place*, chap. 1.

21. *Pen and Picture sketches of the City by the Sea: Atlantic City, The Popular Seaside Resort*, 1874, available at the Historical Society of Pennsylvania Archives, 3–4.

22. *Pen and Picture sketches of the City by the Sea*, 4.

23. *Pen and Picture sketches of the City by the Sea*, 10–12.

24. King, *Atlantic City as a Winter Sanitarium*, 25.

25. King, *Atlantic City as a Winter Sanitarium*, 30.

26. King, *Atlantic City as a Winter Sanitarium*, 27.

27. Shaffer, *See America First*, esp. chap. 1.

28. Visitors' Register, MSS 6/0013-02, Children's Seashore House Records, 1872–1998, College of Physicians of Philadelphia Historical Medical Library, Philadelphia, Pennsylvania.

29. Sears, *Sacred Places*, chap. 5; Mooney and Reinarz, *Permeable Walls*; Miron, *Prisons, Asylums, and the Public*.

30. Lovett, "'Fitter Families for Future Firesides.'" These events were often held in conjunction with Better Babies contests. Crnic, "Better Babies"; Stern, "Making Better Babies," 121–52; Pearson, "'Infantile Specimens.'"

31. Crnic and Connolly, "'They Can't Help Getting Well Here.'" On baby incubator displays—one of which could be found on Atlantic City's boardwalk, see J. Baker, *Machine in the Nursery*, 88–105; Golden, *Babies Made Us Modern*; and B. Hansen, "America's First Medical Breakthrough."

32. Miron, *Prisons, Asylums, and the Public*.

33. "The Children's Seashore House," *Philadelphia Inquirer*, July 3, 1880.

34. *CSH Annual Report*, 1899, 9–10.

35. *CSH Annual Report*, 1875, 13–15.

36. *CSH Annual Report*, 1875, 14.

37. Adams et al., "Kids in the Atrium"; Sloane, "'Not Designed Merely to Heal.'"

38. *Atlantic City and County, New Jersey, Biographically Illustrated.*

39. Brown, *Inventing New England*, 90.

40. Brown, *Inventing New England*, chap. 3. One visitor to Wesleyan Grove even noted the prevalence and visibility of women's housework in these cottage communities.

41. Brown, *Inventing New England.*

42. *CSH Annual Report*, 1894, 11.

43. *CSH Annual Report*, 1902, 12.

44. *CSH Annual Report*, 1902, 12.

45. *Pen and Picture sketches of the City by the Sea*, 17.

46. *Pen and Picture sketches of the City by the Sea*, 18–19.

47. *Pen and Picture sketches of the City by the Sea*, 17.

48. Packard, *Sea-Air and Sea-Bathing*, 10.

49. Packard, *Sea-Air and Sea-Bathing*, 52–53.

50. Packard, *Sea-Air and Sea-Bathing*, 41.

51. Packard, *Sea-Air and Sea-Bathing*, 42.

52. Packard, *Sea-Air and Sea-Bathing*, 36.

53. Packard, *Sea-Air and Sea-Bathing*, 118–19.

54. Packard, *Sea-Air and Sea-Bathing*, 117.

55. *Atlantic City and County, New Jersey, Biographically Illustrated*, 106; Simon, *Boardwalk of Dreams*, 23–24.

56. Funnell, *By the Beautiful Sea*, 18–19.

57. Bryant Simon also provides a similar account and analysis of rolling chairs in his book; see Simon, *Boardwalk of Dreams*, 23–24.

58. Gay J. Talese, "Famous Rolling Chairs beside the Sea," *New York Times*, February 21, 1954.

59. Simon, *Boardwalk of Dreams.*

60. Talese, "Famous Rolling Chairs beside the Sea."

61. Talese, "Famous Rolling Chairs beside the Sea."

62. James B. Howard, Hub-Guard for Wheels, US Patent 753,264, filed June 26, 1903, and issued March 1, 1904.

63. "Atlantic City Season; Gorgeous Private Rolling Chairs the Prevailing Fad," *New York Times*, March 22, 1903.

64. "Atlantic City Season; Gorgeous Private Rolling Chairs the Prevailing Fad."

65. "Roller Chair Rally: Suffragists Plan Novel Parade for Atlantic City," *Washington Post*, June 22, 1913.

66. Parallels exist between the political use of roller chairs and the ways in which women used bicycles as political and social tools; see Neejer, "Bicycle Girls."

67. "Seaside Women Smoke. Puff Cigarettes in Rolling Chairs at Atlantic City. Shock Sedate Boardwalkers," *Washington Post*, June 22, 1915.

68. Quotation from Simon, *Boardwalk of Dreams*, 23–24.

69. Funnell, *By the Beautiful Sea*, 135.

70. Ovington, *City of Robust Health*.

71. Ovington, *City of Robust Health*.

72. Ovington, *City of Robust Health*.

73. Kasson, *Amusing the Million*.

FOUR *How Working-Class Mothers Shaped the Shore*

1. *CSH Annual Report*, 1875, 13.

2. Bennett, "Children's Seashore House [part 1]," 124–25. Bennett also wrote a second article with the same title that was published in the next issue of the *Medical and Surgical Reporter*.

3. Rates could vary, but in 1888 the *CSH Annual Report* recorded a charge of three dollars for a mother with one child, and each additional child was another dollar.

4. Parascandola and Crnic, "Coney Island Babies."

5. Aron, *Working at Play*.

6. One exception is Schlichting, *New York Recentered*. More representative of this trend in the literature is Carr, *Topography of Wellness*.

7. Kathy Peiss's work on Coney Island is a notable exception; see Peiss, *Cheap Amusements*.

8. Bernstein, "Health Activism from the Bottom Up."

9. Simon, *Boardwalk of Dreams*; Kasson, *Amusing the Million*; Peiss, *Cheap Amusements*.

10. Peiss, *Cheap Amusements*.

11. Brown, *Inventing New England*.

12. "Summer Resorts of the Poor," *Daily Graphic*, August 11, 1881.

13. "Summer Resorts of the Poor."

14. Meckel, *Save the Babies*.

15. Obladen, "From Swill Milk to Certified Milk," 81.

16. Meckel, *Save the Babies*, 66–69.

17. Meckel, *Save the Babies*.

18. Hoy, *Chasing Dirt*.

19. DeNoyelles, "'Letting in the Light.'"

20. Kiechle, *Smell Detectives*.

21. Lathrop, *Baby Saving Campaigns*; Meckel, *Save the Babies*.

22. *CSH Annual Report*, 1891, 4; *CSH Annual Report*, 1875, 14.

23. *CSH Annual Report*, 1875, 14.

24. *CSH Annual Report*, 1885, 7–8.

25. *CSH Annual Report*, 1899, 7–8.

26. *CSH Annual Report*, 1875, 8.

27. *CSH Annual Report*, 1881, 10.

28. *CSH Annual Report*, 1886, 7. The babies died later at the hospital.

29. *CSH Annual Report*, 1886, 7.

30. Stainthorpe's first name appears in the 1900 Census for Wilkes-Barre Ward 3, Luzerne, Pennsylvania, Roll 1436, page 5A, accessed at Ancestry.com.

31. According to the 1900 Census, the Stainthorpe family emigrated from England in 1898.

32. "Grateful Woman Praises Children's Seashore House: Read about the Institution in the Inquirer and Returns Thanks," *Philadelphia Inquirer*, August 25, 1901.

33. "Grateful Woman Praises Children's Seashore House."

34. Stainthorpe, September 2, 1901, Patient Register—Cottages, 1901–4, MSS 6/0013-02, Children's Seashore House Records. Amy was readmitted to the cottages with her grandmother on September 2 but was entered in the logbook with the admissions from September 6, 1901; she is listed as patient no. 1423. Her disease remained "rickets," and her result was listed as "improved."

35. "Grateful Woman Praises Children's Seashore House." Confirming information is found Helen Stainthorpe, August 7, 1901, Patient Register—1901–4, MSS 6/0013-02, Children's Seashore House Records.

36. "Grateful Woman Praises Children's Seashore House."

37. *CSH Annual Report*, 1908, 11.

38. Condran and Murphy, "Defining and Managing Infant Mortality"; Meckel, *Save the Babies*.

39. Oates, August 22, 1916, Patient Register—Cottages, MSS 6/0013-02, Children's Seashore House Records. Oates returned annually for several years. Her admissions dates include August 25, 1917, August 2, 1918, August 16, 1919, and August 24, 1920.

40. Rosenberg, *Care of Strangers*; Brandt and Sloane, "Of Beds and Benches"; Sloane, "'Not Designed Merely to Heal.'" On hospitals in the twentieth century, see Stevens, *In Sickness and in Wealth*.

41. Lederer, "Orphans as Guinea Pigs," 102.

42. Theiss, "Least of These."

43. Theiss, "Least of These," 546.

44. James, "Gospel of Relaxation"; Call, *Power through Repose*.

45. *CSH Annual Report*, 1899, 7–8.

46. The Barbara Bates Center for the Study of the History of Nursing, School of Nursing, University of Pennsylvania, has the Starr Centre records in its archives.

47. These two women's families are listed in 1919 as "Frugole" and in 1920 as "Frugoli." Given their first names and the names and ages of their children, it is clear that the families are the same. See Frugole, July 24, 1919, Patient Register—Cottages 1920–24; and Frugoli, July 8, 1920, Patient Register—Cottages 1920–24, both in MSS 6/0013-02, Children's Seashore House Records.

48. Stockman, July 28, 1919, Patient Register—Cottages 1915–19, MSS 6/0013-02, Children's Seashore House Records.

49. Steer, August 22, 1919, Patient Register—Cottages 1915–19, MSS 6/0013-02, Children's Seashore House Records.

50. Steer, August 22, 1919, Patient Register—Cottages 1915–19, MSS 6/0013-02, Children's Seashore House Records.

51. Stockman, Steer, and Brown, July 26, 1920, Patient Register—Cottages 1920–24, MSS 6/0013-02, Children's Seashore House Records.

52. This number is likely an underestimate. There are a number of families who came to the hospital after having been referred by the same Philadelphia-based organizations or institutions, some of which, like the Starr Centre Association, were neighborhood based.

53. See, for instance, Harty, August 25, 1919, Patient Register—Cottages 1915–19, MSS 6/0013-02, Children's Seashore House Records. David Brady and Warren Harty were both eight years old, and admission documents indicated both were "well."

54. Pollack, "Childhood We Have Lost."

55. Adams and Burke, "'Not a Shack in the Woods.'"

56. Edwards, July 1, 1924, Patient Register—Cottages 1920–24, MSS 6/0013-02, Children's Seashore House Records.

57. *CSH Annual Report*, 1909, 12.

58. June 18, 1925, Patient Register—Cottages, June 1925–July 1930, MSS 6/0013-02, Children's Seashore House Records.

59. August 1, 1922, Patient Register—Cottages, 1920–24, MSS 6/0013-02, Children's Seashore House Records.

60. August 7, 1923, Patient Register—Cottages, 1920–24, MSS 6/0013-02, Children's Seashore House Records.

61. Katz, *In the Shadow of the Poorhouse*.

62. *CSH Annual Report*, 1887, 7.

63. *CSH Annual Report*, 1909, 12.

64. *CSH Annual Report*, 1909, 12.

65. Marsh, July 15, 1924, Patient Register—Cottages, 1920–24, MSS 6/0013-02, Children's Seashore House Records.

66. Cepresso, June 18, 1925, Patient Register—Cottages, June 1925–July 1930, MSS 6/0013-02, Children's Seashore House Records.

67. *CSH Annual Report*, 1882, 13. This phrase was often repeated in the annual reports as the institution's objective.

68. Speiser, June 15, 1926, Patient Register—Cottages, June 1925–July 1930, MSS 6/0013-02, Children's Seashore House Records.

69. Wiltse, *Contested Waters*.

70. While this analysis contradicts what some historians have documented about

the class- and race-based dimensions of health care, nurses' actions at the Children's Seashore House align with other histories of public health interventions in this time period, such as urban swimming pools, where race was a secondary factor to class. Wiltse, *Contested Waters.*

71. Bennett, "Children's Seashore House [part 1]," 127.

72. See Waber, July 14, 1925, Patient Register—Cottages, June 1925–July 1930, MSS 6/0013-02, Children's Seashore House Records. On the family who left early due to the food, see Ferri, August 13, 1925, Patient Register—Cottages, June 1925–July 1930, MSS 6/0013-02, Children's Seashore House Records.

73. Hebron, June 16, 1925, Patient Register—Cottages, June 1925–July 1930, MSS 6/0013-02, Children's Seashore House Records.

74. James, "Gospel of Relaxation"; Call, *Power through Repose*; Schuster, "Personalizing Illness and Modernity."

FIVE *Pediatric Patients at the Beach*

1. Alcott, *Little Women*, 275–76.

2. Alcott, *Little Women*, 379.

3. Hope, *Bobbsey Twins at the Seashore*; Thorndyke, *Honey Bunch.*

4. M. Williams, *Velveteen Rabbit.*

5. Stilgoe, *Alongshore*, 340–42.

6. The Episcopal Church of the Ascension in New York City sold the painting in 1981. At the time of the sale, a church warden observed that people either loved or hated it. Laurie Johnston and Robert Mcg. Thomas Jr., "Notes on People: Church to Sell a Painting That Is Both Loved and Hated," *New York Times*, May 11, 1981.

7. "Sorolla Highlights \ Sad Inheritance! 1899," National Gallery of Ireland, 2019, https://www.nationalgallery.ie/art-and-artists/exhibitions/past-exhibitions/sorolla-spanish-master-light/sorolla-highlights-sad.

8. "A 'Distinctly Vulgar Scene' at Coney," Ephemeral New York, August 22, 2014, https://ephemeralnewyork.wordpress.com/2014/08/22/a-distinctly-vulgar-scene-at-coney-island/.

9. Duane et al., *Children's Table.*

10. This methodology is highlighted by others, including Fuentes, *Dispossessed Lives.*

11. Gutman and De Coninck-Smith, *Designing Modern Childhoods*; Marten, "Childhood Studies and History."

12. Mergen, "Children and Nature in History."

13. Paris, *Children's Nature*; S. Miller, *Growing Girls*; Macleod, *Building Character in the American Boy*; MacDonald, *Sons of the Empire.*

14. Zelizer, *Pricing the Priceless Child.*

15. Vanderbeck, "Inner-City Children, Country Summers"; Riney-Kehrberg, *Nature of Childhood.*

16. On the history of childhood and ideas about it, see Clement, *Growing Pains*; Macleod, *Age of the Child*; and Mintz, *Huck's Raft*.

17. Holt, *Diseases of Infancy and Childhood*, 670.

18. Holt, *Diseases of Infancy and Childhood*, 670.

19. Holt, *Diseases of Infancy and Childhood*, 264–65.

20. HUP Ward G, November 1921, 2.

21. HUP Ward G, March 1922.

22. *CSH Annual Report*, 1910, 16.

23. *CSH Annual Report*, 1910, 16.

24. Heith, July 23, 1901, Patient Register—1901–4, MSS 6/0013-02, Children's Seashore House Records.

25. Young; Ziers; Brautigare; Williamson; Johnson; July 23, 1901, Patient Register—1901–4, MSS 6/0013-02, Children's Seashore House Records.

26. Young; Ziers; Brautigare; Williamson; Johnson; July 23, 1901, Patient Register—1901–4, MSS 6/0013-02, Children's Seashore House Records.

27. *CSH Annual Report*, 1914, 10. The schedule and dinner experiences may have varied over time, but these specifics were recorded in the annual reports of the Children's Seashore House.

28. *CSH Annual Report*, 1875, 14.

29. *CSH Annual Report*, 1912, 16.

30. Young; Ziers; Brautigare; Williamson; Johnson; July 23, 1901, Patient Register—1901–4, MSS 6/0013-02, Children's Seashore House Records.

31. Reeves and Shaw, *Children of Craig-Y-Nos*.

32. S. Miller, *Growing Girls*.

33. *CSH Annual Report*, 1913, 25. "Thalasso-therapy" is a term for ocean bathing.

34. *CSH Annual Report*, 1898, 27.

35. *CSH Annual Report*, 1917, 17.

36. MacDonald, *Sons of the Empire*.

37. Bederman, *Manliness and Civilization*.

38. *CSH Annual Report*, 1897, 8–9.

39. *CSH Annual Report*, 1897, 8.

40. *CSH Annual Report*, 1905, 14–15.

41. *CSH Annual Report*, 1905, 14–15.

42. *CSH Annual Report*, 1897, 8–9.

43. Crnic and Connolly, "'They Can't Help Getting Well Here.'"

44. "The Story of 'Smiling Joe' a Boy Whose Cheerfulness in Affliction Has Opened the Door of Hope to Thousands," *World's Events*, July 1909, 6; "$250,000 Raised by a Sick Boy's Smile," *New York Times*, May 2, 1909.

45. "Story of 'Smiling Joe.'"

46. "How a Photograph of a Helpless Crippled Tot Built a Hospital," *Washington Post*, December 3, 1911.

47. "Roosevelt Surprises Coney and Big Fleet." Sea Breeze, and Roosevelt's visit to it, are also detailed in Crnic and Connolly, "'They Can't Help Getting Well Here.'"

48. "A Cheerful View of a Serious Situation," *Gunter's Magazine*, vol. 8, 1906, author's collection.

49. "Cheerful View of a Serious Situation." It seems that the Association for Improving the Condition of the Poor was unaware of the Children's Seashore House.

50. Newspapers reported various numbers for New York City children who had nonpulmonary tuberculosis. Most claimed between four thousand to forty-five hundred, and at least one mentioned that upwards of five thousand children suffered from the condition.

51. "Cheerful View of a Serious Situation" (original emphasis).

52. Quoted in "Cheerful View of a Serious Situation."

53. This is roughly equivalent to $4.2 million in 2022.

54. "City Decides to Buy Two Seaside Parks," *New York Times*, July 28, 1911.

55. "$250,000 Raised by a Sick Boy's Smile."

56. "Seaside Sanitarium Would Save Life," *New York Times*, November 30, 1909.

57. "$250,000 Raised by a Sick Boy's Smile."

58. "Seaside Sanitarium Would Save Life."

59. "How a Photograph of a Helpless Crippled Tot Built a Hospital," *Washington Post*, December 3, 1911.

60. Levander and Singley, *American Child*, 3–4.

61. Howard Gershenfeld, "Five Year Diary," January 1, 1940, private collection (referred to hereafter in the following format: Howard G, "Five Year Diary," date). I am deeply grateful to Howard's children, who agreed to let me read their father's diary and encouraged me to use his full name. Howard had wanted to be an author and see his name in print. I hope I have honored his legacy.

62. "This Just In: USC Also Is a 1939 Champion," *Washington Post*, July 28, 2004.

63. Howard G, "Five Year Diary," January 19, 1940.

64. Howard G, "Five Year Diary," February 3, 1940.

65. Howard G, "Five Year Diary," January 15, 1940.

66. Howard G, "Five Year Diary," February 13, 1940.

67. Howard G, "Five Year Diary," March 5, 1940.

68. Howard G, "Five Year Diary," January 23, 1940.

69. Howard G, "Five Year Diary," January 25, 1940.

70. Howard G, "Five Year Diary," January 22, 1940.

71. Howard G, "Five Year Diary," January 10, 1940.

72. Howard G, "Five Year Diary," January 31, 1940.

73. Howard G, "Five Year Diary," February 1, 1940.

74. Howard G, "Five Year Diary," February 4, 1940.

75. Howard G, "Five Year Diary," February 12, 1940.

76. Howard G, "Five Year Diary," February 4, 1940.

77. Edward John Hudak, "Memories of Seashore House: For Kids, It Was More than 'Marine Medication,'" *Philadelphia Daily News*, July 12, 1990.

78. Hudak, "Memories of Seashore House."

79. Hudak, "Memories of Seashore House."

80. Hudak, "Memories of Seashore House."

81. Hudak, "Memories of Seashore House."

82. Hudak, "Memories of Seashore House."

83. *CSH Annual Report*, 1914, 11.

84. Cynthia Connolly, email message to the author, December 19, 2018.

SIX *Doctor Sun and Technologies of Nature*

1. Boston Floating Hospital, *Thirty Second Annual Report*, 1925, 32–33, accessed at Countway Library, Harvard Medical School.

2. Howell, *Technology in the Hospital*.

3. Carter, "Leagues of Sunshine"; Freund, *American Sunshine*, 94; Sadar, "Healthful Ambience of Vitaglass"; Woloshyn, "*Le Pays du Soleil*."

4. One example of a natural-light mimicking machine was the ozone generator; see Kiechle, "'Health Is Wealth,'" 792. For a more contemporary discussions of biomimicry, see Fisch, "Nature of Biomimicry."

5. Rollier, *Heliotherapy*, 24.

6. Rollier, *Heliotherapy*, 157. At Leysin, in the Swiss Alps, patients with cardiac conditions wore an additional white cloth over their chests to protect their thoracic cavities.

7. Brannan, "Heliotherapy in Tuberculosis of the Bones and Joints," 153. Both Rollier and Brannan presented at the 1908 International Congress of Tuberculosis conference, held in Washington, DC. Rollier, "La cure d'altitude et la cure solaire de la tuberculose," 301.

8. Brannan, "Heliotherapy in Tuberculosis of the Bones and Joints," 157.

9. Brannan, "Heliotherapy in Tuberculosis of the Bones and Joints," 156.

10. Brannan, "Heliotherapy in Tuberculosis of the Bones and Joints," 153. See also Austin, "Heliotherapy for Tuberculous Children."

11. Bunker, "Light and Life," 683.

12. Rollier, "Heliotherapy," 817.

13. Woloshyn, "Patients Rebuilt."

14. Gauvain, "Discussion on the General Principles of Treatment in Tuberculosis Disease," 880.

15. Gauvain, "Discussion on the General Principles of Treatment in Tuberculosis Disease," 879.

16. Gauvain, "Discussion on the General Principles of Treatment in Tuberculosis Disease," 879.

17. Woloshyn, "Patients Rebuilt." For more on rickets, see Semba, "Impact of Improved Nutrition on Disease Prevention," 164–65; Warren, "Gardener in the Machine"; and Apple, *Vitamania*.

18. Brannan, "Heliotherapy in Tuberculosis of the Bones and Joints," 157.

19. Russell and Russell, *Ultra-Violet Radiation and Actinotherapy*, 20.

20. Carter, "Leagues of Sunshine," 99–109; Gauvain, "Discussion on the General Principles of Treatment in Tuberculous Disease."

21. Downes and Blunt, "Researches on the Effect of Light," 496–97.

22. Clemensen, "Brief Review of Finsen's Phototherapy."

23. Russell and Russell, *Ultra-Violet Radiation and Actinotherapy*, 16.

24. Schamberg, "Present Status of Phototherapy," 543.

25. Clemensen, "Brief Review of Finsen's Phototherapy," 920.

26. "The Nobel Prize in Physiology or Medicine 1903," Nobelprize.org, accessed January 21, 2013, http://www.nobelprize.org/nobel_prizes/medicine/laureates/1903/.

27. Schamberg, "Present Status of Phototherapy," 543.

28. Willard, "Sunshine and Fresh Air," 156.

29. Schamberg, "Present Status of Phototherapy," 548–49.

30. Bie, "Remarks on Finsen's Phototherapy," 827. The description of Finsen's lamp comes from two sources: Bie, "Remarks on Finsen's Phototherapy," 826–27; and Clemensen, "Brief Review of Finsen's Phototherapy," 923–24.

31. Bie, "Remarks on Finsen's Phototherapy."

32. Schamberg, "Present Status of Phototherapy," 548.

33. Schamberg, "Present Status of Phototherapy," 543.

34. Willard, "Sunshine and Fresh Air," 155.

35. Bie, "Remarks on Finsen's Phototherapy," 829.

36. Bie, "Remarks on Finsen's Phototherapy," 829.

37. Russell, "Heliotherapy and Actinotherapy," 167. Vitaglass was glass that allowed UV rays to penetrate. Sadar, "The Healthful Ambience of Vitaglass."

38. Russell, "Heliotherapy and Actinotherapy," 167.

39. Warren, *Starved for Light*.

40. Semba, "Impact of Improved Nutrition on Disease Prevention," 164; Connolly, *Saving Sickly Children*, 49. Connolly also documents the shock of the medical community at discovering that tuberculosis exposure was so widespread among children. Unlike rickets, tuberculosis was understood by physicians to be primarily a disease of adulthood.

41. As quoted in Tisdall, "Etiology of Rickets," 938.

42. Hess and Unger, "Use of the Carbon Arc Light in the Prevention and Cure of Rickets," 1598.

43. Hess and Unger, "Use of the Carbon Arc Light in the Prevention and Cure of Rickets," 1596.

44. Freund, *American Sunshine*, 38–40.

45. Chick, "Study of Rickets in Vienna," 41–51.

46. Freund, *American Sunshine*, 38–40; Rajakumar and Thomas, "Reemerging Nutritional Rickets."

47. Warren, "Gardener in the Machine."

48. Tisdall, "Deficiency Diseases of Children," 906.

49. Bunker and Harris, "Precise Evaluation of Light Therapy in Experimental Rickets," 1287.

50. Tracy, "Heliotherapy Tent," 451–52.

51. Schwartz, "Application of Radiation in the Modern Hospital," 693.

52. Tom Condon, "Last Hope for a Shoreline Landmark," *CT Mirror*, August 12, 2016, https://ctmirror.org/2016/08/12/last-hope-for-a-shoreline-landmark/.

53. Tisdall, "Sunlight and Health," 694–95.

54. Russell, "Heliotherapy and Actinotherapy," 167. As British physician and artificial light champion W. Kerr Russell noted, it was not possible or desirable to send every urban patient to the seashore or mountains.

55. Schwartz, "Application of Radiation in the Modern Hospital."

56. This image appears both in Gamgee, *Artificial Light Treatment of Children*; and Russell and Russell, *Ultra-Violet Radiation and Actinotherapy*.

57. Woloshyn, *Kiss of Light*, 24.

58. Schwartz, "Application of Radiation in the Modern Hospital," 696.

59. Other scholars, including Margarete Sandelowski, have traced the ways in which medical technologies such as thermometers have been "passed down" from physicians to nurses and the public, resulting in the technology's loss of status as an exclusive medical device. Sandelowski, *Devices and Desires*.

60. Andress and Evans, *Health and Success*, 117.

61. Andress and Evans, *Health and Success*, 119–20.

62. Andress and Evans, *Health and Success*, 116.

63. Andress and Evans, *Health and Success*, 116.

64. Andress and Evans, *Health and Success*, 120.

65. Andress and Evans, *Health and Success*, 117.

66. Andress and Evans, *Health and Success*, 119–20.

67. Harris, "Heliotherapy in Surgical Tuberculosis," 691.

68. "Value of Sunlight in the Home," *Good Housekeeping* 27, no. 3 (1892): 72.

69. *Sunlight for Babies* (Children's Bureau, US Department of Labor, 1926), 2. Author's collection.

70. *Sunlight for Babies*, 5–6. Historians have detailed how governmental officials increasingly targeted mothers via health campaigns; see Ladd-Taylor, *Raising a Baby the Government Way*; and Lindenmeyer, *Right to Childhood*.

71. Freund, *American Sunshine*, 106.

72. *Sunlight for Babies*, 8. For more on the history of sunbathing in America and its associations with health, see Freund, *American Sunshine*.

73. Romano, "Dark Side of the Sun"; Freund, *American Sunshine*, 116.

74. "Value of Sunlight in the Home"; Smuts, *Science in the Service of Children*; Apple, *Perfect Motherhood*.

75. S. Baker, "Importance of Good Health," 35. On the idea of the plasticity of children, see Crnic, "Better Babies."

76. Austin, "Heliotherapy for Tuberculous Children," 839.

77. *Sunlight for Babies*, 1931, 4.

78. Freund, *American Sunshine*, 116.

79. Day, "98.6"; Connolly, *Children and Drug Safety*.

80. Egan, "Boston Floating Hospital," 401.

81. Le Boutillier, "Sea-Water Treatment, Given by Subcutaneous Injection," 26–28.

Conclusion

1. "About Cystic Fibrosis," Cystic Fibrosis Foundation, accessed February 28, 2024, https://www.cff.org/.

2. Peggy Peck, "Studies Look to Sea for Cystic Fibrosis Treatment," CNN, January 19, 2006, http://www.cnn.com/2006/HEALTH/conditions/01/18/cf.saltwater/index.html (no longer available).

3. The authors explained that "in vitro data suggested that sustained hydration of airway surfaces was responsible for the sustained improvement in mucus clearance, whereas inhibition of osmotically driven water transport by amiloride accounted for the observed loss of clinical benefit." Donaldson et al., "Mucus Clearance and Lung Function in Cystic Fibrosis with Hypertonic Saline," 241.

4. Elkins et al., "Controlled Trial of Long-Term Inhaled Hypertonic Saline," 229; Donaldson et al., "Mucus Clearance and Lung Function in Cystic Fibrosis with Hypertonic Saline."

5. Peck, "Studies Look to Sea for Cystic Fibrosis Treatment."

6. Azeen Ghorayshi, "Read an Excerpt from a Memoir of a Young Woman Who Died of a Superbug Infection: *Salt in My Soul* Is a New Memoir about a Young Woman's Life with Cystic Fibrosis," Buzzfeed, March 11, 2019, https://www.buzzfeednews.com/article/azeenghorayshi/salt-in-my-soul-cystic-fibrosis-memoir. The article the father read was Rosenfeld et al., "Inhaled Hypertonic Saline in Infants and Toddlers with Cystic Fibrosis."

7. On the rise of randomized controlled trials as the gold standard of medical investigation, see Marks, *Progress of Experiment*.

8. Physicians concluded that inhaling saline had a "moderate" certainty of benefit to patients with CF. Mogayzel et al., "Cystic Fibrosis Pulmonary Guidelines."

9. Feudtner, *Bittersweet*.

10. Oshinsky, *Polio*; Schupmann, "Human Experimentation in Public Schools."

11. Stafford, "Prescribed Vacations."

12. Stafford, "Prescribed Vacations."

13. Singer, "Medically Supervised Vacational Migrations," 904.

14. Singer, "Medically Supervised Vacational Migrations," 904–5.

15. Singer, "Medically Supervised Vacational Migrations," 906. According to Google Scholar, Singer's article has only been cited twice, including once by Singer himself.

16. Singer, "Medically Supervised Vacational Migrations," 905.

17. Mitman, *Breathing Space*; Lewis, *Chasing the Cure in New Mexico*; Abel, *Suffering in the Land of Sunshine.*

18. According to a press release, the hospital planned to continue to provide intensive and specialty care services. "End of an Era: The Closing of Tufts Children's Hospital, Putting Inpatient Pediatric Care in Context," Tufts University School of Medicine, Center for Health Systems and Policy, April 8, 2022, https://sites.tufts.edu/chsp/2022/04/08/end-of-an-era-the-closing-of-tufts-childrens-hospital-putting-inpatient-pediatric-care-in-context/.

19. Louv, *Last Child in the Woods.*

20. "Author Richard Louv Honored with the 50th Audubon Medal," National Audubon Society, January 24, 2008, https://www.audubon.org/news/author-richard-louv-honored-50th-audubon-medal.

21. Timothy, online customer review of *Last Child in the Woods*, Amazon.com, August, 26, 2017, https://www.amazon.com/Last-Child-Woods-Children-Nature-Deficit/product-reviews/156512605X/ref=cm_cr_dp_d_show_all_btm?ie,=UTF8&reviewerType=all_reviews.

22. Joyce, online customer review of *Last Child in the Woods*, Amazon.com, November 13, 2012, https://www.amazon.com/Last-Child-Woods-Children-Nature-Deficitproduct-reviews/156512605X/ref=cm_cr_dp_d_show_all_btm?ie,=UTF8&reviewerType=all_reviews.

23. Gretchen Reynolds, "How Walking in Nature Changes the Brain," *New York Times*, July 22, 2015.

24. Reynolds, "How Walking in Nature Changes the Brain."

25. This was the number as of February 27, 2024. Bratman et al., "Benefits of Nature Experience."

26. Frumkin et al., "Nature Contact and Human Health."

27. "Parkrx: About," ParkRx, accessed February 28, 2024, https://www.parkrx.org/about.

28. Ginia Bellafante, "Schools Beat Earlier Plagues with Outdoor Classes. We Should Too," *New York Times*, July 17, 2020.

29. M. Hansen, Jones, and Tocchini, "Shinrin-yoku (Forest Bathing) and Nature Therapy."

30. Nutsford et al., "Residential Exposure to Visible Blue Space," 70. The authors do not distinguish between naturally occurring and constructed lakes. See also Völker

and Kistemann, "Impact of Blue Space on Human Health and Well-Being"; Foley and Kistemann, "Blue Space Geographies"; White et al., "Blue Space, Health, and Well-Being"; and Britton et al., "Blue Care."

31. Jacobsen, "Against Sunscreen Absolutism."

32. Markevych et al., "Exploring Pathways Linking Greenspace to Health."

33. Nash, "Fruits of Ill-Health."

34. Shanahan et al., "Health Benefits from Nature Experiences Depend on Dose"; Seresinhe, Preis, and Moat, "Quantifying the Impact of Scenic Environments on Health."

35. My colleague Michelle Kondo and I also make this argument in Crnic and Kondo, "Nature Rx."

36. Murphy, *Sick Building Syndrome and the Problem of Uncertainty.*

37. Smith, *Salt in My Soul,* 101.

BIBLIOGRAPHY

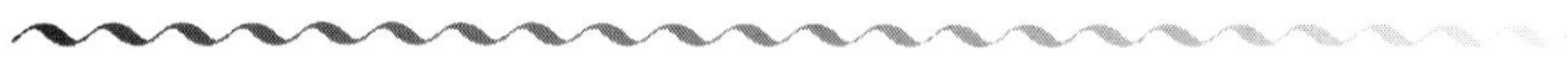

Abel, Emily. *Suffering in the Land of Sunshine: A Los Angeles Illness Narrative*. New Brunswick, NJ: Rutgers University Press, 2006.

Abrams, Laura S., and Laura Curran. "Between Women: Gender and Social Work in Historical Perspective." *Social Service Review* 78, no. 3 (2004): 429–46.

Adams, Annmarie. *Architecture in the Family Way: Doctors, Houses, and Women, 1870–1900*. Montreal: McGill-Queen's University Press, 1996.

Adams, Annmarie, and Stacie Burke. "'Not a Shack in the Woods': Architecture for Tuberculosis in Muskoka and Toronto." *Canadian Bulletin of Medical History* 23, no. 2 (2006): 429–55.

Adams, Annmarie, David Theodore, Ellie Goldenberg, Coralee McLaren, and Patricia McKeever. "Kids in the Atrium: Comparing Architectural Intentions and Children's Experiences in a Pediatric Hospital Lobby." *Social Science and Medicine* 70, no. 5 (2010): 658–67.

Alcott, Louisa May. *Little Women*. 1868–69. New York: Signet Classics, 2012.

Andress, James Mace, and William Augustus Evans. *Health and Success*. Boston: Ginn and Company, 1925.

Antonovsky, Aaron. "The Salutogenic Model as a Theory to Guide Health Promotion." *Health Promotion International* 11, no. 1 (1996): 11–18.

Apple, Rima D. *Mothers and Medicine: A Social History of Infant Feeding, 1890–1950*. Madison: University of Wisconsin Press, 1987.

———. *Perfect Motherhood: Science and Childrearing in America*. New Brunswick, NJ: Rutgers University Press, 2006.

———. *Vitamania: Vitamins in American Culture*. New Brunswick, NJ: Rutgers University Press, 1996.

Aron, Cindy. *Working at Play: A History of Vacations in the United States*. New York: Oxford University Press, 2001.

Atkins, Thomas Benjamin. *Out of the Cradle into the World: Or Self Education through Play*. Columbus, OH: Sterling, 1895.

Atlantic City and County, New Jersey, Biographically Illustrated: A Short Biography, Illustrated by Portraits, of Prominent Residents of Atlantic County and the Famous Summer and Winter Resort, Celebration Throughout America Atlantic City. Philadelphia: Alfred M. Slocum, 1899.

Austin, Gertrude. "Heliotherapy for Tuberculous Children." *The Child* (1912): 839–45.

Baker, Jeffrey P. *The Machine in the Nursery: Incubator Technology and the Origins of Newborn Intensive Care*. Baltimore: Johns Hopkins University Press, 1996.

Baker, S. Josephine. "The Importance of Good Health." *Woman's Home Companion*, January 1914.

Bakker, Nelleke. "Before Ritalin: Children and Neurasthenia in the Netherlands." *Paedagogica Historica* 46, no. 3 (2010): 383–401.

Bates, Barbara. *Bargaining for Life: A Social History of Tuberculosis 1876–1938*. Philadelphia: University of Pennsylvania Press, 1992.

Bean, William B. "Walter Reed and the Ordeal of Human Experiments." *Bulletin of the History of Medicine* 51, no. 1 (1977): 75–92.

Bederman, Gail. *Manliness and Civilization: A Cultural History of Gender and Race in the United States, 1880–1917*. Chicago: University of Chicago Press, 1995.

Bennett, William D. "The Children's Seashore House, at Atlantic City, and Its Clinical Teachings in Regard to the Value of the Seashore as a Resort for Sick Children [part 1]." *Medical and Surgical Reporter* 38, no. 7 (February 16, 1878): 124–27.

———. "The Children's Seashore House, at Atlantic City, and Its Clinical Teachings in Regard to the Value of the Seashore as a Resort for Sick Children [part 2]." *Medical and Surgical Reporter* 38, no. 8 (February 23, 1878): 141–46.

Benson, Etienne S. *Surroundings: A History of Environments and Environmentalisms*. Chicago: University of Chicago Press, 2020.

Bernstein, Shana. "Health Activism from the Bottom Up: Progressive Era Immigrant Chicagoans' Views on Germ Theory, Environmental Health, and Class Inequality." *Journal of the Gilded Age and Progressive Era* 17, no. 2 (2018): 317–44.

Berridge, Virginia, and Martin Gorsky, eds. *Environment, Health and History*. London: Palgrave Macmillan, 2012.

Bie, Valdemar. "Remarks on Finsen's Phototherapy." *British Medical Journal* 2, no. 2022 (September 30, 1899): 825–30.

Bornside, George H. "Jaime Ferran and Preventive Inoculation Against Cholera." *Bulletin of the History of Medicine* 55, no. 4 (1981): 516–32.

Borsay, Anne, and Pamela Dale, eds. *Disabled Children: Contested Caring, 1850–1979*. New York: Routledge, 2012.

Boyer, Paul S. *Urban Masses and Moral Order in America, 1820–1920*. Cambridge, MA: Harvard University Press, 1992.

Brandt, Allan M., and David C. Sloane. "Of Beds and Benches: Building the Modern American Hospital." In *The Architecture of Science*, edited by Peter Galison and Emily Thompson, 281–308. Cambridge, MA: MIT Press, 1999.

Brannan, John W. "Heliotherapy in Tuberculosis of the Bones and Joints." *Transactions of the American Climatological and Clinical Association* 30 (1914): 149–64.

———. "The Seashore and Fresh Air Treatment at Sea Breeze Hospital." In *Transactions of the Sixth International Congress on Tuberculosis*, 2:682–700.

Bratman, Gregory N., Gretchen C. Daily, Benjamin J. Levy, and James J. Gross. "The Benefits of Nature Experience: Improved Affect and Cognition." *Landscape and Urban Planning* 138 (2015): 41–50.

Breckinridge, Sophonisba P., ed. *The Child in the City: A Series of Papers Presented at the Conference Held during the Chicago Child Welfare Exhibit*. Chicago: Department of Social Investigation, Chicago School of Civics and Philanthropy, 1912.

Britton, Easkey, Gesche Kindermann, Christine Domegan, and Caitriona Carlin. "Blue Care: A Systematic Review of Blue Space Interventions for Health and Wellbeing." *Health Promotion International* 35, no. 1 (2020): 50–69.

Brochard, André Théodore. *Sea-Air and Sea-Bathing for Children and Invalids: Their Properties, Use, & Mode of Employment*. London: Longman, Green, Longman, Roberts & Green, 1865.

Brooks-Gunn, Jeanne, and Anna Duncan Johnson. "G. Stanley Hall's Contribution to Science, Practice, and Policy: The Child Study, Parent Education, and Child Welfare Movements." *History of Psychology* 9, no. 3 (2006): 247–58.

Brosco, Jeffrey Paul. "Sin or Folly: Child and Community Health in Philadelphia, 1900–1930." PhD diss., University of Pennsylvania, 1994.

———. "Weight Charts and Well-Child Care: How the Pediatrician Became the Expert in Child Health." *Archives of Pediatrics and Adolescent Medicine* 155, no. 12 (2001): 1385–89.

Brown, Dona. *Inventing New England: Regional Tourism in the Nineteenth Century*. Washington, DC: Smithsonian Institution Press, 1995.

Bunker, John W. M. "Light and Life." *American Journal of Public Health* 16, no. 7 (1926): 676–86.

Bunker, John W. M., and Robert S. Harris. "The Precise Evaluation of Light Therapy in Experimental Rickets." *American Journal of Public Health and the Nation's Health* 20, no. 12 (1930): 1287–92.

Byrom, Brad. "The Progressive Movement and the Child with Physical Disabilities." In *Children with Disabilities in America: A Historical Handbook and Guide*, edited by Philip L. Safford and Elizabeth J. Safford, 49–64. Westport, CT: Greenwood Press, 2006.

Call, Annie Payson. *Power through Repose*. Boston: Little, Brown, 1902.

Carboni, Gian Piero. "The Enigma of Pacini's *Vibrio cholerae* Discovery." *Journal of Medical Microbiology* 70, no. 11 (2021). https://doi.org/10.1099/jmm.0.001450.

Carr, Sara Jensen. *The Topography of Wellness: How Health and Disease Shaped the American Landscape*. Charlottesville: University of Virginia Press, 2021.

Carter, Simon. "Leagues of Sunshine: Sunlight, Health and the Environment." In Berridge and Gorsky, *Environment, Health and History*, 94–112.

Cavallo, Dominick. *Muscles and Morals: Organized Playgrounds and Urban Reform, 1880–1920*. Philadelphia: University of Pennsylvania Press, 1981.

Chick, Harriette. "Study of Rickets in Vienna 1919–1922." *Medical History* 20, no. 1 (1976): 41–51.

Clemensen, P. C. "A Brief Review of Finsen's Phototherapy." *Journal of the American Medical Association* 38, no. 15 (1902): 919–25.

Clement, Priscilla Ferguson. *Growing Pains: Children in the Industrial Age, 1850–1890.* New York: Twayne, 1997.

Condran, Gretchen A., and Jennifer Murphy. "Defining and Managing Infant Mortality: A Case Study of Philadelphia, 1870–1920." *Social Science History* 32, no. 4 (2008): 473–513.

Connolly, Cynthia A. *Children and Drug Safety: Balancing Risk and Protection in Twentieth-Century America.* New Brunswick, NJ: Rutgers University Press, 2018.

———. *Saving Sickly Children: The Tuberculosis Preventorium in American Life, 1909–1970.* New Brunswick, NJ: Rutgers University Press, 2008.

Cooter, Roger. *Surgery and Society in Peace and War: Orthopaedics and the Organization of Modern Medicine, 1880–1948.* London: Palgrave Macmillan, 1993.

Corbin, Alain. *The Lure of the Sea: The Discovery of the Seaside in the Western World, 1750–1840.* Berkeley: University of California Press, 1994.

Cowan, Ruth Schwartz. *More Work for Mother: The Ironies of Household Technology from the Open Hearth to the Microwave.* New York: Basic Books, 1983.

Cranz, Galen. *The Politics of Park Design: A History of Urban Parks in America.* Cambridge, MA: MIT Press, 1982.

Crnic, Meghan. "Better Babies: Social Engineering for 'a Better Nation, a Better World.'" *Endeavour* 33, no. 1 (2009): 12–17.

Crnic, Meghan, and Cynthia Connolly. "'They Can't Help Getting Well Here': Seaside Hospitals for Children in the United States: 1872–1917." *Journal of the History of Childhood and Youth* 2, no. 2 (2009): 220–33.

Crnic, Meghan, and Michelle C. Kondo. "Nature Rx: Reemergence of Pediatric Nature-Based Therapeutic Programs from the Late 19th and Early 20th Centuries." *American Journal of Public Health* 109, no. 10 (2019): 1371–78. https://doi.org/10.2105/ajph.2019.305204.

Cronon, William. *Nature's Metropolis: Chicago and the Great West.* New York: Norton, 1992.

———. "The Trouble with Wilderness: Or, Getting Back to the Wrong Nature." *Environmental History* 1, no. 1 (1996): 7–28.

Day, Deanna. "98.6: Fevers, Fertility, and the Patient Labor of American Medicine." PhD diss., University of Pennsylvania, 2014.

deNoyelles, Adrienne. "'Letting in the Light': Jacob Riis's Crusade for Breathing Spaces on the Lower East Side." *Journal of Urban History* 46, no. 4 (2020): 775–93.

Donaldson, Scott H., William D. Bennett, Kirby L. Zeman, Michael R. Knowles, Robert Tarran, and Richard C. Boucher. "Mucus Clearance and Lung Function in

Cystic Fibrosis with Hypertonic Saline." *New England Journal of Medicine* 354, no. 3 (2006): 241–50.

Donegan, Jane B. *Hydropathic Highway to Health: Women and Water-Cure in Antebellum America*. New York: Greenwood Press, 1986.

Downes, Arthur, and Thomas Blunt. "Researches on the Effect of Light upon Bacteria and Other Organisms." *Proceedings of the Royal Society of London* 26, no. 179–84 (1878): 488–500.

Duane, Anna Mae, ed. *The Children's Table: Childhood Studies and the Humanities*. Athens: University of Georgia Press, 2013.

Dye, Nancy Schrom, and Daniel Blake Smith. "Mother Love and Infant Death, 1750–1920." *Journal of American History* 73, no. 2 (1986): 329–53.

Dyl, Joanna L. "The War on Rats versus the Right to Keep Chickens: Plague and the Paving of San Francisco, 1907–1908." In *The Nature of Cities: Culture, Landscape and Urban Space*, edited by Andrew C. Isenberg, 38–61. Rochester, NY: University of Rochester Press, 2006.

Egan, Sara "The Boston Floating Hospital." *AJN: The American Journal of Nursing* 32, no. 4 (1932): 401–2.

Ehrenreich, John. *The Altruistic Imagination: A History of Social Work and Social Policy in the United States*. Ithaca: Cornell University Press, 1985.

Elkins, Mark R., Michael Robinson, Barbara R. Rose, Colin Harbour, Carmel P. Moriarty, Guy B. Marks, Elena G. Belousova, Wei Xuan, and Peter T. P. Bye. "A Controlled Trial of Long-Term Inhaled Hypertonic Saline in Patients with Cystic Fibrosis." *New England Journal of Medicine* 354, no. 3 (2006): 229–40.

Fairchild, Amy L. "Policies of Inclusion: Immigrants, Disease, Dependency, and American Immigration Policy at the Dawn and Dusk of the 20th Century." *American Journal of Public Health* 94, no. 4 (2004): 528–39.

Feudtner, John Christopher. *Bittersweet: Diabetes, Insulin, and the Transformation of Illness*. Chapel Hill: University of North Carolina Press, 2003.

Fisch, Michael. "The Nature of Biomimicry: Toward a Novel Technological Culture." *Science, Technology, & Human Values* 42, no. 5 (2017): 795–821.

Fisher, Colin. *Urban Green: Nature, Recreation, and the Working Class in Industrial Chicago*. Chapel Hill: University of North Carolina Press, 2015.

Flanagan, Maureen A. "The City Profitable, the City Livable: Environmental Policy, Gender, and Power in Chicago in the 1910s." *Journal of Urban History* 22, no. 2 (1996): 163–90.

Foley, Ronan, and Thomas Kistemann. "Blue Space Geographies: Enabling Health in Place." *Health & Place* 35 (September 2015): 157–65.

Freund, Daniel. *American Sunshine: Diseases of Darkness and the Quest for Natural Light*. Chicago: University of Chicago Press, 2012.

Frumkin, Howard, Gregory N. Bratman, Sara Jo Breslow, Bobby Cochran, Peter H.

Kahn Jr., Joshua J. Lawler, Phillip S. Levin, et al. "Nature Contact and Human Health: A Research Agenda." *Environmental Health Perspectives* 125, no. 7 (2017): 075001–18.

Fuentes, Marisa J. *Dispossessed Lives: Enslaved Women, Violence, and the Archive*. Philadelphia: University of Pennsylvania Press, 2016.

Funnell, Charles. *By the Beautiful Sea: The Rise and High Times of That Great American Resort, Atlantic City*. New Brunswick, NJ: Rutgers University Press, 1983.

Gamgee, Katherine M. L. *The Artificial Light Treatment of Children in Rickets, Anaemia and Malnutrition*. London: Lewis, 1927.

Gauvain, Henry. "Discussion on the General Principles of Treatment in Tuberculous Disease of the Bones and Joints in Children." *British Medical Journal* 2, no. 3178 (1921): 876–84.

———. "The Hastings Popular Lecture on Sun, Air, and Sea Bathing in Health and Disease." *British Medical Journal* 1, no. 3764 (1933): 57–61.

———. "Sea Bathing in the Treatment of Surgical Tuberculosis." *British Medical Journal* 2, no. 3909 (1935): 1087–90.

Golden, Janet. *Babies Made Us Modern: How Infants Brought America into the Twentieth Century*. Cambridge: Cambridge University Press, 2018.

———. "Children's Health: Caregivers and Sites of Care." In Golden, Merkel, and Prescott, *Children and Youth in Sickness and in Health*, 67–84.

Golden, Janet, Richard Meckel, and Heather Munro Prescott, eds. *Children and Youth in Sickness and in Health*. Westport, CT: Greenwood Press, 2004.

Grant, Julia. *Raising Baby by the Book: The Education of American Mothers*. New Haven: Yale University Press, 1998.

Greene, Ann Norton. *Horses at Work: Harnessing Power in Industrial America*. Cambridge, MA: Harvard University Press, 2008.

Grover, Kathryn, ed. *Hard at Play: Leisure in America, 1840–1940*. Amherst: University of Massachusetts Press, 1992.

Guarneri, Julia. "Changing Strategies for Child Welfare, Enduring Beliefs about Childhood: The Fresh Air Fund, 1877–1926." *Journal of the Gilded Age and Progressive Era* 11, no. 1 (2012): 27–70.

Gutman, Marta. *A City for Children: Women, Architecture, and the Charitable Landscapes of Oakland, 1850–1950*. Chicago: University of Chicago Press, 2014.

Gutman, Marta, and Ning De Coninck-Smith, eds. *Designing Modern Childhoods: History, Space, and the Material Culture of Children*. New Brunswick, NJ: Rutgers University Press, 2008.

Hall, Granville Stanley. *The Story of a Sand-Pile*. New York: E. L. Kellogg & Company, 1897.

Halpern, Sydney A. *American Pediatrics: The Social Dynamics of Professionalism, 1880–1980*. Berkeley: University of California Press, 1988.

Hammond, Roland. "Heliotherapy (of Rollier) as an Adjunct in the Treatment of Bone Disease." *Journal of Bone and Joint Surgery* s2-11, no. 2 (1913): 269–75.

———. "The Seashore Treatment of Osteomyelitis." *Journal of Bone and Joint Surgery* s2-10, no. 4 (1913): 569–83.

———. "Treatment of Bone Tuberculosis at the Crawford Allen Hospital (Seashore Branch of the Rhode Island Hospital)." *Boston Medical and Surgical Journal* 165, no. 2 (1911): 49–51.

Hammonds, Evelynn Maxine. *Childhood's Deadly Scourge: The Campaign to Control Diphtheria in New York City, 1880–1930*. Baltimore: Johns Hopkins University Press, 1999.

Hansen, Bert. "America's First Medical Breakthrough: How Popular Excitement about a French Rabies Cure in 1885 Raised New Expectations for Medical Progress." *American Historical Review* 103, no. 2 (1998): 373–418.

Hansen, Margaret M., Reo Jones, and Kirsten Tocchini. "Shinrin-Yoku (Forest Bathing) and Nature Therapy: A State-of-the-Art Review." *International Journal of Environmental Research and Public Health* 14, no. 8 (2017): 851.

Harris, R. I. "Heliotherapy in Surgical Tuberculosis." *American Journal of Public Health* 16, no. 7 (1926): 687–94.

Hays, Samuel P. *Conservation and the Gospel of Efficiency: The Progressive Conservation Movement, 1890–1920*. Pittsburgh: University of Pittsburgh Press, 1999.

Herbert, Amanda E. "Gender and the Spa: Space, Sociability and Self at British Health Spas, 1640–1714." *Journal of Social History* 43, no. 2 (Winter 2009): 361–83.

Hess, Alfred F., and Lester J. Unger. "Use of the Carbon Arc Light in the Prevention and Cure of Rickets." *Journal of the American Medical Association* 78, no. 21 (1922): 1596–98.

Hill, Leonard, and J. Argyll Campbell, with the cooperation of Sir Henry Gauvain. "Metabolism of Children Undergoing Open-Air Treatment, Heliotherapy and Balneotherapy." *British Medical Journal* 1, no. 3191 (February 25, 1922): 301–3.

Hinsdale, Guy. *Atmospheric Air in Relation to Tuberculosis*. Washington, DC: Smithsonian Institution, 1914.

Hofstadter, Richard. *The Age of Reform: From Bryan to FDR*. New York: Vintage Books, 1955.

Holt, Luther Emmett. *The Diseases of Infancy and Childhood*. New York: D. Appleton, 1897.

Hope, Laura Lee. *The Bobbsey Twins at the Seashore*. New York: Grosset & Dunlap, 1907.

Howell, Joel D. *Technology in the Hospital: Transforming Patient Care in the Early Twentieth Century*. Baltimore: Johns Hopkins University Press, 1995.

Hoy, Suellen. *Chasing Dirt: The American Pursuit of Cleanliness*. New York: Oxford University Press, 1995.

Jacobsen, Rowan. "Against Sunscreen Absolutism." *The Atlantic*, May 10, 2024. https://www.theatlantic.com/magazine/archive/2024/06/sun-exposure-health-benefits/678205/.

Jain, Sarah S. Lochlann. " 'Dangerous Instrumentality': The Bystander as Subject in Automobility." *Cultural Anthropology* 19, no. 1 (2004): 61–94.

James, William. "The Gospel of Relaxation." In *Talks to Teachers on Psychology*, edited by William James, 199–228. New York: H. Holt and Co., 1899.

Jones, Karen R. "'The Lungs of the City': Green Space, Public Health and Bodily Metaphor in the Landscape of Urban Park History." *Environment and History* 24, no. 1 (2018): 39–58.

Kasson, John F. *Amusing the Million: Coney Island at the Turn of the Century*. New York: Hill and Wang, 1978.

Katz, Michael B. *In the Shadow of the Poorhouse: A Social History of Welfare in America*. New York: Basic Books, 1996.

Kelley, Florence. "The Street Trader under Illinois Law." In Breckinridge, *Child in the City*, 290–301.

Kevles, Daniel J. *In the Name of Eugenics: Genetics and the Uses of Human Heredity*. Cambridge, MA: Harvard University Press, 1995.

Kiechle, Melanie A. "'Health Is Wealth': Valuing Health in the Nineteenth-Century United States." *Journal of Social History* 54, no. 3 (2021): 775–98.

———. "'Nature's Great Disinfectant, Prophylactic, Curative, Stimulant, and Sedative': Ozone Generators and Personal Provisions for Health." Paper presented at the annual meeting of the Society for the History of Technology, Portland, Maine, October 10–13, 2013.

———. "Navigating by Nose: Fresh Air, Stench Nuisance, and the Urban Environment, 1840–1880." *Journal of Urban History* 42, no. 4 (2016): 753–71.

———. *Smell Detectives: An Olfactory History of Nineteenth-Century Urban America*. Seattle: University of Washington Press, 2017.

King, John T. *Atlantic City as a Winter Sanitarium: Its Geology, Climate, and Isothermal Relations and Its Sanitary Effect Upon Diseases and Invalids*. Baltimore: B. H. James & Co., Fine Book and Job Printers, 1881. https://babel.hathitrust.org/cgi/pt?id=loc.ark:/13960/t1vd72g16.

Koven, Seth. "Remembering and Dismemberment: Crippled Children, Wounded Soldiers, and the Great War in Great Britain." *American Historical Review* 99, no. 4 (1994): 1167–1202.

Kraut, Alan M. *Silent Travelers: Germs, Genes, and the "Immigrant Menace."* Baltimore: Johns Hopkins University Press, 1995.

Ladd-Taylor, Molly. *Raising a Baby the Government Way: Mothers' Letters to the Children's Bureau, 1915–1932*. New Brunswick, NJ: Rutgers University Press, 1986.

Ladd-Taylor, Molly, and Lauri Umansky, eds. *"Bad" Mothers: The Politics of Blame in Twentieth-Century America*. New York: New York University Press, 1998.

LaFay, Elaine. "Afflictions of the Tropics' Brink: Medicine, Meteorology, and the Cultivation of Place in the Antebellum Gulf South." PhD diss., University of Pennsylvania, 2019.

Lathrop, Julia C. *Baby-Saving Campaigns: A Preliminary Report on What American Cities Are Doing to Prevent Infant Mortality*. Washington, DC: US Department of Labor, Children's Bureau, 1913.

Lawrence, Christopher, and George Weisz, eds. *Greater than the Parts: Holism in Biomedicine, 1920–1950*. New York: Oxford University Press, 1998.

Lears, T. Jackson. *Rebirth of a Nation: The Making of Modern America, 1877–1920*. New York: HarperCollins, 2009.

Leavitt, Judith Walzer. *The Healthiest City: Milwaukee and the Politics of Health Reform*. Madison: University of Wisconsin Press, 1996.

———. *Typhoid Mary: Captive to the Public's Health*. Boston: Beacon Press, 1996.

Le Boutillier, Theodore. "Sea-Water Treatment, Given by Subcutaneous Injection with the Results Obtained in Children." *Journal of the American Medical Association* 54, no. 1 (1910): 26–28. https://doi.org/10.1001/jama.1910.92550270001001h.

Lederer, Susan E. "Orphans as Guinea Pigs: American Children and Medical Experimenters, 1890–1930." In *In the Name of the Child: Health and Welfare, 1880–1940*, edited by Roger Cooter, 96–123. London: Routledge, 1992.

Levander, Caroline Field, and Carol J. Singley, eds. *The American Child: A Cultural Studies Reader*. New Brunswick, NJ: Rutgers University Press, 2003.

Lewis, Nancy Owen. *Chasing the Cure in New Mexico: Tuberculosis and the Quest for Health*. Santa Fe: Museum of New Mexico Press, 2016.

Lewis, R. "The Beach at Atlantic City." *Harper's Weekly*, August 30, 1873.

Lindenmeyer, Kriste. *A Right to Childhood: The US Children's Bureau and Child Welfare, 1912–46*. Urbana: University of Illinois Press, 1997.

Livingston, Julie. *Debility and the Moral Imagination in Botswana*. Bloomington: Indiana University Press, 2005.

Linker, Beth. "On the Borderland of Medical and Disability History: A Survey of the Fields." *Bulletin of the History of Medicine* 87, no. 4 (2013): 499–535.

———. *War's Waste: Rehabilitation in World War I America*. Chicago: University of Chicago Press, 2011.

Lombardo, Paul A. *Three Generations, No Imbeciles: Eugenics, the Supreme Court, and Buck V. Bell*. Baltimore: Johns Hopkins University Press, 2022.

Louv, Richard. *Last Child in the Woods: Saving Our Children from Nature Deficit Disorder*. Chapel Hill: Algonquin Books of Chapel Hill, 2008.

Lovett, Laura L. "'Fitter Families for Future Firesides': Florence Sherbon and Popular Eugenics." *Public Historian* 29, no. 3 (2007): 69–85.

MacDonald, Robert. *Sons of the Empire: The Frontier and Boy Scouts Movement, 1890–1918*. Toronto: University of Toronto Press, 1993.

Macleod, David I. *The Age of the Child: Children in America, 1890–1920*. New York: Twayne, 1998.

———. *Building Character in the American Boy: The Boy Scouts, YMCA, and Their Forerunners, 1870–1920*. Madison: University of Wisconsin Press, 1983.

Madrigal, Alexis C. "Aghast over Beijing's Air Pollution? This Was Pittsburgh Not That Long Ago." *The Atlantic*, January 16, 2013. https://www.theatlantic.com/technology/archive/2013/01/aghast-over-beijings-air-pollution-this-was-pittsburgh-not-that-long-ago/267237/.

Markevych, Iana, Julia Schoierer, Terry Hartig, Alexandra Chudnovsky, Perry Hystad, Angel M. Dzhambov, Sjerp de Vries, et al. "Exploring Pathways Linking Greenspace to Health: Theoretical and Methodological Guidance." *Environmental Research* 158 (October 2017): 301–17. https://doi.org//10.1016/j.envres.2017.06.028.

Markowitz, Gerald, and David Rosner. *Lead Wars: The Politics of Science and the Fate of America's Children*. Berkeley: University of California Press; New York: Milband Memorial Fund, 2013.

Marks, Harry M. *The Progress of Experiment: Science and Therapeutic Reform in the United States, 1900–1990*. Cambridge: Cambridge University Press, 1997.

Marten, James. "Childhood Studies and History: Catching a Culture in High Relief." In Duane, *Children's Table*, 52–67.

McNeur, Catherine. *Taming Manhattan: Environmental Battles in the Antebellum City*. Cambridge, MA: Harvard University Press, 2014.

Meckel, Richard A. *Save the Babies: American Public Health Reform and the Prevention of Infant Mortality, 1850–1929*. Baltimore: Johns Hopkins University Press, 1990.

Melosi, Martin V. *The Sanitary City: Environmental Services in Urban America from Colonial Times to the Present*. Pittsburgh: University of Pittsburgh Press, 2008.

Mergen, Bernard. "Children and Nature in History." *Environmental History* 8, no. 4 (2003): 643–69.

Miller, Albert H. "The Seashore Treatment of the Tubercular Arthritis of Children." *Boston Medical and Surgical Journal* 157, no. 20 (1907): 659–61.

Miller, D. J. Milton. "Memoir of Dr. William Henry Bennett." *Transactions of the College of Physicians of Philadelphia* 42 (1920): 187–94.

Miller, Susan A. *Growing Girls: The Natural Origins of Girls' Organizations in America*. New Brunswick, NJ: Rutgers University Press, 2007.

Minardi, Margot. "The Boston Inoculation Controversy of 1721–1722: An Incident in the History of Race." *William and Mary Quarterly* 61, no. 1 (2004): 47–76.

Mintz, Steven. *Huck's Raft: A History of American Childhood*. Cambridge, MA: Harvard University Press, 2004.

Miron, Janet. *Prisons, Asylums, and the Public: Institutional Visiting in the Nineteenth Century*. Toronto: University of Toronto Press, 2011.

Mitman, Gregg. *Breathing Space: How Allergies Shape Our Lives and Landscapes*. New Haven: Yale University Press, 2007.

———. "Hay Fever Holiday: Health, Leisure, and Place in Gilded-Age America." *Bulletin of the History of Medicine* 77, no. 3 (2003): 600–635.

Mogayzel, Peter J., Jr., Edward T. Naureckas, Karen A. Robinson, Gary Mueller, Denis Hadjiliadis, Jeffrey B. Hoag, Lisa Lubsch, et al. "Cystic Fibrosis Pulmonary Guidelines: Chronic Medications for Maintenance of Lung Health." *American Journal of Respiratory and Critical Care Medicine* 187, no. 7 (2013): 680–89.

Mooney, Graham, and Jonathan Reinarz, eds. *Permeable Walls: Historical Perspectives on Hospital and Asylum Visiting*. New York: Rodopi, 2009.

Muir, John. *The Yosemite*. New York: The Century Co., 1912.

Munns, David P. D. "'Not by a Decree of Fate': Ellen Richards, Euthenics, and the Environment in the Progressive Era." *Journal of the History of Biology* 56, no. 3 (2023): 525–57.

Murphy, Michelle. *Sick Building Syndrome and the Problem of Uncertainty: Environmental Politics, Technoscience, and Women Workers*. Durham, NC: Duke University Press, 2006.

Nasaw, David. *Children of the City: At Work and at Play*. New York: Doubleday, 1985.

Nash, Linda. "The Fruits of Ill-Health: Pesticides and Workers' Bodies in Post–World War II California." *Osiris*, 2nd ser., 19 (2004): 203–19.

———. *Inescapable Ecologies: A History of Environment, Disease, and Knowledge*. Berkeley: University of California Press, 2006.

Neejer, Christine. "The Bicycle Girls: American Wheelwomen and Everyday Activism in the Late Nineteenth Century." PhD diss., Michigan State University, 2016.

Nelson, Marie C., and Staffan Förhammar. "Swedish Seaside Sanatoria in the Beginning of the Twentieth Century." *Journal of the History of Childhood and Youth* 2, no. 2 (2009): 249–66.

Nissenbaum, Stephen. *Sex, Diet, and Debility in Jacksonian America: Sylvester Graham and Health Reform*. Westport, CT: Greenwood Press, 1980.

Nutsford, Daniel, Amber L. Pearson, Simon Kingham, and Femke Reitsma. "Residential Exposure to Visible Blue Space (but Not Green Space) Associated with Lower Psychological Distress in a Capital City." *Health & Place* 39 (May 2016): 70–78.

Obladen, Michael. "From Swill Milk to Certified Milk: Progress in Cow's Milk Quality in the 19th Century." *Annals of Nutrition and Metabolism* 64, no. 1 (2014): 80–87.

Ogle, Maureen. *All the Modern Conveniences: American Household Plumbing, 1840–1890*. Baltimore: Johns Hopkins University Press, 1996.

Oliver, George. "The Therapeutics of the Sea-Side: With Special Reference to the North-East Coast." *British Medical Journal* 2, no. 516 (November 19, 1870): 550–51.

Oshinsky, David M. *Polio: An American Story*. Oxford: Oxford University Press, 2005.

Ott, Katherine. *Fevered Lives: Tuberculosis in American Culture since 1870*. Cambridge, MA: Harvard University Press, 1996.

Ovington, Earle. *The City of Robust Health*. Atlantic City: Chamber of Commerce, 1918.

Packard, John Hooker. *Sea-Air and Sea-Bathing*. Philadelphia: Blakiston, 1880.

Palm, Theobald. "The Geographical Distributions and Etiology of Rickets." *The Practitioner* 45 (1890): 270–79, 321–42.

Parascandola, John, and Meghan Crnic. "Coney Island Babies: Children's Aid Societies and Health Homes at Coney Island." *New York History* 104, no. 2 (2023): 383–405.

Paris, Leslie. *Children's Nature: The Rise of the American Summer Camp*. New York: New York University Press, 2008.

Pearson, Susan J. "'Infantile Specimens': Showing Babies in Nineteenth-Century America." *Journal of Social History* 42, no. 2 (Winter 2008): 341–70.

Peiss, Kathy. *Cheap Amusements: Working Women and Leisure in New York City, 1880–1920*. Philadelphia: Temple University Press, 1986.

Peña, Carolyn Thomas de la. "Recharging at the Fordyce: Confronting the Machine and Nature in the Modern Bath." *Technology and Culture* 40, no. 4 (1999): 746–69.

Pernick, Martin S. "Politics, Parties, and Pestilence: Epidemic Yellow Fever in Philadelphia and the Rise of the First Party System." *William and Mary Quarterly: A Magazine of Early American History* 29, no. 4 (1972): 559–86.

Philadelphia Railroad. *Atlantic City, N.J., the Great American Sea-Side Resort: A Brief Sketch of Its Resources, Advantages and Railway Facilities*. Philadelphia: Press of Allen, Lane and Scott, 1894. https://hdl.handle.net/2027/njp.32101072334038.

Plater, M. "Tonic for Body or Soul: Fresh Air for Poor Children in Progressive Era New York City." *Journal of Urban History* 49, no. 4 (2023): 865–90.

Pollack, Eunice G. "The Childhood We Have Lost: When Siblings Were Caregivers, 1900–1970." *Journal of Social History* 36, no. 1 (2002): 31–61.

Porter, Roy. *The Greatest Benefit to Mankind: A Medical History of Humanity*. New York: Norton, 1998.

———, ed. "The Medical History of Waters and Spas." Supplement no. 10, *Medical History* (1990).

Rajakumar, Kumaravel, and Stephen B. Thomas. "Reemerging Nutritional Rickets: A Historical Perspective." *Archives of Pediatric Adolescent Medicine* 159, no. 4 (2005): 335–41. https://doi.org/10.1001/archpedi.159.4.335.

Reber, Vera Blinn. "Poor, Ill, and Sometimes Abandoned: Tubercular Children in Buenos Aires, 1880–1920." *Journal of Family History* 27, no. 2 (2002): 128–49.

Reed, Boardman. "Diseased Conditions for Which Sea Air Is of Doubtful Benefit." *Transactions of the Fourth Annual Meeting of the American Climatological Association*, 42–45. Philadelphia: Printed for the association, 1887.

———. "The Effects of Sea Air upon Diseases of the Respiratory Organs, Including a Study of the Influence upon Health of Changes in the Atmospheric Pressure." *Transactions of the First Annual Meeting of the American Climatological Association*, 51–58. New York: D. Appleton, 1884.

Reeves, Carole, and Ann Shaw. *The Children of Craig-Y-Nos: Life in a Welsh Tuberculosis Sanatorium, 1922–1959*. London: Wellcome Trust Centre for the History of Medicine at UCL, 2009.

Richards, Ellen Henrietta. *Euthenics, the Science of Controllable Environment: A Plea for Better Living Conditions as a First Step toward Higher Human Efficiency*. Boston: Whitcomb & Barrows, 1910.

Riney-Kehrberg, Pamela. *The Nature of Childhood: An Environmental History of Growing Up in America since 1865*. Lawrence: University Press of Kansas, 2014.

Ritchie, Robert C. *The Lure of the Beach: A Global History*. Oakland: University of California Press, 2021.

Robison, John. "Ocean Climates: Their Effects and the Cases They Benefit." *Journal of the American Medical Association* 36, no. 18 (1901): 1244–45.

Rogers, Naomi. *Dirt and Disease: Polio before FDR*. New Brunswick, NJ: Rutgers University Press, 1992.

Rollier, Auguste. *Heliotherapy*. London: Henry Frowde and Hodder & Stoughton, 1923.

———. "Heliotherapy: Its Therapeutic, Prophylactic and Social Value." *American Journal of Nursing* 27, no. 10 (1927): 815–23.

———. "La cure d'altitude et la cure solaire de la tuberculose." In *Transactions of the Sixth International Congress on Tuberculosis*, 2:301–2.

Romano, Sally Dunne. "The Dark Side of the Sun: Skin Cancer, Sunscreen, and Risk in Twentieth-Century America." PhD diss., Yale University, 2006.

Rosen, George. "Disease, Debility, and Death." In *The Victorian City*, Volume 2, edited by Jim Dyos and Michael Wolff, 625–67. New York: Routledge, 1999.

Rosenberg, Charles E. *The Care of Strangers: The Rise of America's Hospital System*. New York: Basic Books, 1987.

———. *The Cholera Years: The United States in 1832, 1849, and 1866*. Chicago: University of Chicago Press, 1987.

———. "The Tyranny of Diagnosis: Specific Entities and Individual Experience." *Milbank Quarterly* 80, no. 2 (2002): 237–60.

Rosenfeld, Margaret, Stephanie Davis, Lyndia Brumback, Stephen Daniel, Ron Rowbotham, Robin Johnson, Sharon McNamara, et al. "Inhaled Hypertonic Saline in Infants and Toddlers with Cystic Fibrosis: Short-Term Tolerability, Adherence, and Safety." *Pediatric Pulmonology* 46, no. 7 (2011): 666–71.

Rothman, Sheila M. *Living in the Shadow of Death: Tuberculosis and the Social Experience of Illness in American History*. New York: Basic Books, 1995.

Russell, Eleanor Hilda Wylam, and William Kerr Russell. *Ultra-Violet Radiation and Actinotherapy*. New York: William Wood, 1927.

Russell, W. Kerr. "Heliotherapy and Actinotherapy." *British Medical Journal* 1, no. 3395 (1926): 167.

Sadar, John. "The Healthful Ambience of Vitaglass: Light, Glass and the Curative Environment." *Architectural Research Quarterly* 12, no. 3–4 (2008): 269–81.

Sandelowski, Margarete. *Devices and Desires: Gender, Technology, and American Nursing*. Chapel Hill: University of North Carolina Press, 2000.

Schamberg, Jay Frank. "The Present Status of Phototherapy." *Journal of the American Medical Association* 49, no. 7 (1907): 543–50.

Schlichting, Kara Murphy. *New York Recentered: Building the Metropolis from the Shore.* Chicago: University of Chicago Press, 2019.

Schupmann, Will D. "Human Experimentation in Public Schools: How Schools Served as Sites of Vaccine Trials in the 20th Century." *American Journal of Public Health* 108, no. 8 (2018): 1015–22.

Schuster, David G. *Neurasthenic Nation: America's Search for Health, Happiness, and Comfort, 1869–1920.* New Brunswick, NJ: Rutgers University Press, 2011.

———. "Personalizing Illness and Modernity: S. Weir Mitchell, Literary Women, and Neurasthenia, 1870–1914." *Bulletin of the History of Medicine* 79, no. 4 (2005): 695–722.

Schwartz, R. Plato. "The Application of Radiation in the Modern Hospital." *AJN: The American Journal of Nursing* 26, no. 9 (1926): 691–96.

Schweik, Susan M. *The Ugly Laws: Disability in Public.* New York: New York University Press, 2009.

Sears, John F. *Sacred Places: American Tourist Attractions in the Nineteenth Century.* New York: Oxford University Press, 1989.

Sellers, Christopher. "Thoreau's Body: Towards an Embodied Environmental History." *Environmental History* 4, no. 4 (1999): 486–514.

———. "To Place or Not to Place: Toward an Environmental History of Modern Medicine." *Bulletin of the History of Medicine* 92, no. 1 (2018): 1–45.

Semba, Richard. "The Impact of Improved Nutrition on Disease Prevention." In *Silent Victories: The History and Practice of Public Health in Twentieth-Century America,* edited by John W. Ward and Christian Warren, 163–92. Oxford: Oxford University Press, 2007.

Seresinhe, Chanuki Illushka, Tobias Preis, and Helen Susannah Moat. "Quantifying the Impact of Scenic Environments on Health." *Scientific Reports* 5, no. 1 (2015): 16899.

Shaffer, Marguerite Sands. *See America First: Tourism and National Identity, 1880–1940.* Washington, DC: Smithsonian Institution Press, 2001.

Shanahan, Danielle F., Robert Bush, Kevin J. Gaston, Brenda B. Lin, Julie Dean, Elizabeth Barber, and Richard A. Fuller. "Health Benefits from Nature Experiences Depend on Dose." *Scientific Reports* 6, no. 1 (2016): 28551.

Shands, A. R., Jr. "DeForest Willard, Philadelphia's Pioneer Orthopaedic Surgeon (1846–1910)." *Current Practice in Orthopaedic Surgery* 4 (1969): 43–57.

Shearer, Tobin Miller. *Two Weeks Every Summer: Fresh Air Children and the Problem of Race in America.* Ithaca: Cornell University Press, 2017.

Simon, Bryant. *Boardwalk of Dreams: Atlantic City and the Fate of Urban America.* New York: Oxford University Press, 2004.

———. "A Natural History of the Life and Death of a Great American City: Atlantic City, New Jersey, 1850–2000." In *New Jersey's Environments: Past, Present, and Future,* edited by Neil M. Maher, 11–27. New Brunswick, NJ: Rutgers University Press, 2006.

Singer, Charles I. "Medically Supervised Vacational Migrations." *Journal of the American Medical Association* 112, no. 10 (1939): 904–7.

Sloane, David. "'Not Designed Merely to Heal': Women Reformers and the Emergence of Children's Hospitals." *Journal of the Gilded Age and Progressive Era* 4, no. 4 (2005): 331–54.

Smith, Mallory. *Salt in My Soul: An Unfinished Life*. New York: Random House, 2019.

Smuts, Alice Boardman. *Science in the Service of Children, 1893–1935*. New Haven: Yale University Press, 2008.

Snodgrass, Mary Ellen. *The Civil War Era and Reconstruction: An Encyclopedia of Social, Political, Cultural and Economic History*. London: Routledge, 2015.

Spencer-Wood, Suzanne M. "Turn of the Century Women's Organizations, Urban Design, and the Origin of the American Playground Movement." *Landscape Journal* 13, no. 2 (1994): 124–37.

Spirn, Anne Whiston. "Constructing Nature: The Legacy of Frederick Law Olmsted." In *Uncommon Ground: Rethinking the Human Place in Nature*, edited by William Cronon, 91–113. Rev. ed. New York: Norton, 1996.

———. *The Granite Garden: Urban Nature and Human Design*. New York: Basic Books, 1984.

Stafford, Jane. "Prescribed Vacations." *Science News-Letter*, June 1939, 362–64.

Stern, Alexandra Minna. "Making Better Babies: Public Health and Race Betterment in Indiana, 1920–1935." *American Journal of Public Health* 92, no. 5 (2002): 742–52.

Stern, Alexandra Minna, and Howard Markel, eds. *Formative Years: Children's Health in the United States, 1880–2000*. Ann Arbor: University of Michigan Press, 2002.

Stevens, Rosemary. *In Sickness and in Wealth: American Hospitals in the Twentieth Century*. Baltimore: Johns Hopkins University Press, 1999.

Stewart, W. Blair. "Influence of Sea-Air and Sea-Water Baths on Disease." *Journal of the American Medical Association* 35, no. 11 (1900): 678–79.

Stilgoe, John R. *Alongshore*. New Haven: Yale University Press, 1994.

Stradling, David. *Making Mountains: New York City and the Catskills*. Seattle: University of Washington Press, 2007.

———. *Smokestacks and Progressives: Environmentalists, Engineers, and Air Quality in America, 1881–1951*. Baltimore: Johns Hopkins University Press, 1999.

Swanson, Kara W. "Human Milk as Technology and Technologies of Human Milk: Medical Imaginings in the Early Twentieth-Century United States." *WSQ: Women's Studies Quarterly* 37, no. 1 (2009): 20–37.

Tarr, Joel A. *The Search for the Ultimate Sink: Urban Pollution in Historical Perspective*. Akron, OH: University of Akron Press, 1996.

Theiss, Lewis Edwin. "The Least of These: What the Fresh Air Movement Means to the Children of the Slums." *Outing Magazine: The Outdoor Magazine of Human Interest*, no. 54 (August 1909): 538–49.

Thorndyke, Helen Louise *Honey Bunch: Her First Visit to the Seashore*. New York: Grosset and Dunlap, 1924.

Thorsheim, Peter. *Inventing Pollution: Coal, Smoke, and Culture in Britain since 1800*. Athens: Ohio University Press, 2017.

Tisdall, Frederick F. "Deficiency Diseases of Children." *Canadian Medical Association Journal* 15, no. 9 (1925): 904–8.

———. "The Etiology of Rickets." *Canadian Medical Association Journal* 11, no. 12 (1921): 934–43.

———. "Sunlight and Health." *American Journal of Public Health* 16, no. 7 (1926): 694–99.

Tomes, Nancy. *The Gospel of Germs: Men, Women, and the Microbe in American Life*. Cambridge, MA: Harvard University Press, 1999.

Tracy, Margaret. "A Heliotherapy Tent." *American Journal of Nursing* 27, no. 6 (1927): 451–52.

Transactions of the Sixth International Congress on Tuberculosis, Washington, September 28 to October 5, 1908. 6 vols. in 8. Philadelphia: W. F. Fell, 1908.

Valenčius, Conevery Bolton. "Gender and the Economy of Health on the Santa Fe Trail." *Osiris* 19, no. 1 (2004): 79–92.

———. *The Health of the Country: How American Settlers Understood Themselves and Their Land*. New York: Basic Books, 2002.

Vanderbeck, Robert M. "Inner-City Children, Country Summers: Narrating American Childhood and the Geographies of Whiteness." *Environment and Planning* 40, no. 5 (2008): 1132–50.

Vanobbergen, Bruno. "Belgian Sea Hospitals and the Child at Risk: Exploring an Educational Paradox." *Journal of the History of Childhood and Youth* 2, no. 2 (2009): 234–48.

Vanobbergen, Bruno, and Nancy Vansieleghem. "Repairing the Body, Restoring the Soul: The Sea Hospital of the City of Paris in Berck-sur-Mer and the French War on Tuberculosis." *Paedagogica Historica* 46, no. 3 (2010): 325–40.

Vogel, Morris J., and Charles E. Rosenberg, eds. *The Therapeutic Revolution: Essays in the Social History of American Medicine*. Philadelphia: University of Pennsylvania Press, 2017.

Völker, Sebastian, and Thomas Kistemann. "The Impact of Blue Space on Human Health and Well-Being—Salutogenetic Health Effects of Inland Surface Waters: A Review." *International Journal of Hygiene and Environmental Health* 214, no. 6 (2011): 449–60.

Warner, John Harley. *The Therapeutic Perspective: Medical Practice, Knowledge, and Identity in America, 1820–1885*. Princeton: Princeton University Press, 2014.

Warren, Christian. "The Gardener in the Machine: Biotechnological Adaptation for Life Indoors." In Berridge and Gorsky, *Environment, Health and History*, 206–23.

———. *Starved for Light: The Long Shadow of Rickets and Vitamin D Deficiency*. Chicago: University of Chicago Press, 2024.

Weaver, Lawrence T. "In the Balance: Weighing Babies and the Birth of the Infant Welfare Clinic." *Bulletin of the History of Medicine* 84, no. 1 (2010): 30–57.

Weigley, Emma Seifrit. "It Might Have Been Euthenics: The Lake Placid Conferences and the Home Economics Movement." *American Quarterly* 26, no. 1 (1974): 79–96.

Weisz, George. "Spas, Mineral Waters, and Hydrological Science in Twentieth-Century France." *Isis* 92, no. 3 (September 2001). https://doi.org/10.1086/385278.

Whitbeck, B. H. "A Review of the Ten Years' Work at Sea Breeze Hospital for Surgical Tuberculosis." *Journal of Bone and Joint Surgery* s2-14, no. 3 (1916): 119–33.

White, Mathew P., Lewis R. Elliott, Mireia Gascon, Bethany Roberts, and Lora E. Fleming. "Blue Space, Health and Well-Being: A Narrative Overview and Synthesis of Potential Benefits." *Environmental Research* 191 (December 2020): 110169.

Willard, DeForest. "Sunshine and Fresh Air vs. the Finsen Ultra-Violet Rays and the Roentgen Rays in Tuberculosis of the Joints and Bone." *Journal of the American Medical Association* 41, no. 3 (July 18, 1903): 154–58.

Williams, Margery. *The Velveteen Rabbit*. 1922. New York: Doubleday, 1991.

Williams, Raymond. *The Country and the City*. Oxford: Oxford University Press, 1975.

Willoughby, Urmi Engineer. *Yellow Fever, Race, and Ecology in Nineteenth-Century New Orleans*. Baton Rouge: Louisana State University Press, 2017.

Wiltse, Jeff. *Contested Waters: A Social History of Swimming Pools in America*. Chapel Hill: University of North Carolina Press, 2007.

Winpenny, Thomas. "The Engineer as Promoter: Richard B. Osborne, the Camden and Atlantic Railroad, and the Creation of Atlantic City." *Essays in Economic and Business History* 22 (2004): 301–12.

Woloshyn, Tania. *The Kiss of Light: Nursing and Light Therapy in Twentieth Century Britain*. Edited by Natasha McEnroe. London: Florence Nightingale Museum and the Wellcome Trust, 2015.

———. "*Le Pays du Soleil*: The Art of Heliotherapy on the Côte d'Azur." *Social History of Medicine* 26, no. 1 (2013): 74–93.

———. "Patients Rebuilt: Dr Auguste Rollier's Heliotherapeutic Portraits, c. 1903–1944." *Medical Humanities* 39, no. 1 (2013): 38–46.

Worboys, Michael. *Spreading Germs: Diseases, Theories and Medical Practice in Britain, 1865–1900*. Cambridge: Cambridge University Press, 2000.

Wright, David. *SickKids: The History of the Hospital for Sick Children*. Toronto: University of Toronto Press, 2017.

Zelizer, Viviana A. *Pricing the Priceless Child: The Changing Social Value of Children*. Princeton: Princeton University Press, 1994.

Zinguer, Tamar. "The Sandbox: How Women Planted Play in the City." *Material Culture* 54, no. 2 (2022).

Zueblin, Charles. "The City Child at Play." In Breckinridge, *Child in the City*, 443–50.

INDEX

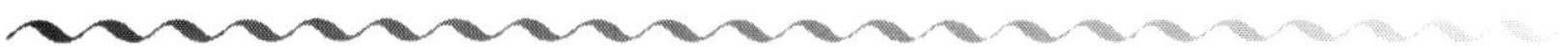

Page numbers in *italic* refer to illustrations.

Alcott, Louisa May: *Little Women*, 97

Andress, J. Mace: *Health and Success*, *138*, 138–39

anthrax, 40

Association for Improving the Condition of the Poor, 26, 80, *113*, 114,

Atlantic City, NJ, 44–45, 58, 60–78; baby incubator exhibits, 39, 66; bathers, *59*; beach, *59*, 62, *63*; boardwalk, 74, 91; rolling chairs, *72*, 73–76. *See also* Children's Seashore House

Atkins, T. Benjamin, 20–21

bacteriology, 57; opsonic index, 49; penicillin, 145; and properties of sunlight, 54, 127, 130

balneotherapy (swimming), xii, 50, 52, 55, 102

bathhouses, 60, 70–71; hot springs at, 26

Beach at Coney Island (Bellows), *99*, 99–100

beachfront hospitals. *See* hospitals

Bellows, George: *Beach at Coney Island*, *99*, 99–100; *Forty-Two Kids*, *100*, 100

Bennett, William H.: and admissions to hospital, 85, 93, 107; and day care, 92–93, 108; and happiness, 105, 121–22; and seashore's rehabilitative properties, 47, 56, 89–90, 105

Blunt, Thomas, 130

Boston: hospitals in, 26, *30*, 31, 33, 123, *125*, 142, 147; park system in, 19; restricted use of beaches in, 20; rickets in, 15; "sand gardens" in, 18, 19; smallpox in, 13

Boston Floating Hospital, 26, *30*, 31, 33, 123, *125*, 142, 147

Brannan, John, 126, 129

Bratman, Gregory, 148–49

Brochard, André, 41, 50

Camden, NJ, 28

camps, summer, 43, 108–11

Central Park (New York City), 20, 61

Chicago: air pollution in, 22; beaches in, 5, 20; population of, 13; sand gardens, 19

child development, 16–17, 103

child mortality, 12–14, 21, 29

children, immigrant, 15, 23–24

Children's Bureau. *See* US Children's Bureau

Children's Seashore House (Atlantic City, NJ), 41, 43–44, 56, 69–70, 104–11, 117–21; buildings, 66–69, *67*, *68*; closure of, 147; mothers and children at, 79–81, 84–94; promotion of, 64–66; sea-bathing at, 50, 51–52; summer camps at, 108–11; sunbathing at, 126; treatment of "debility" by, 42, 43; wintertime care at, 46–47. *See also* Bennett, William H.

cholera, 3, 13, 40

"cholera infantum," 14

Clark, Harriette, 135

class. *See* middle class; upper class; working class

cold-water bathing, 50, 161n70

Coney Island (New York City) , *7*, 7, 31, 32, 77; "baby incubator" shows, 39; Bellows's painting of, *99*, 99–100; "health homes," 80. *See also* Sea Breeze Hospital
Coney Island Sea Salt, *7*, 7
Couney, Martin, 39
COVID-19 pandemic, 149
Crawford Allen Hospital, 47–48, 56; sunbathing at, 54–55, 127
cystic fibrosis (CF), 143–44, 151

"debility," 14, 16, 41–43, 85, 106
diphtheria, 3, 4, 13, 14, 40, 145
Donaldson, Scott, 143–44
Downes, Arthur, 130
Doyle, Arthur Conan, 76

England, 41, 42, 44, 52, 56, 133. *See also* Hayling Island
environmental health, 146, 149. *See also* public health
epidemics, 3, 13, 53; bubonic plague, 13; smallpox, 13; yellow fever, 3, 4, 13
Evans, W. A.: *Health and Success*, *138*, 138–39

Finsen, Niels, 130–33, *132*, 136
"forest bathing," 149
Forty-Two Kids (Bellows), *100*, 100
France, 37, 38, 146–47
Fresh Air Fund, 26, 31

Gauvain, Henry, 52, 56, 127
gender norms, 75, 81
germ theory of disease, 4, 6, 49, 53
Gershenfeld, Howard, 117–21

Hall, G. Stanley, 18, 19, 108
Hammond, Roland, 49, 55
Hayling Island, 52, 56, 127
Health and Success (Andress and Evans), *138*, 138–39
health homes, 2, 31, 80, 84, 88
health resorts, 26, 34, 146–47
heliotherapy, 54–56, *125*, 126–29, *128*, 134–41, 150
Hess, Alfred, 134, 135
Holt, L. Emmett, 103–4
home health conditions, 22–25, 47, 83–84
hospitals: children's, 37–38, 89, 101; in England, 52, 56, 127; in Europe, 37, 42, 147; floating, 26, *30*, 31; in Philadelphia, 25, 42, 147; in Rhode Island, 47–48, 54–55, 56; seashore, 37, 42, 46, 89, 101–2, 129; as tourist attraction, 65; in Waterford, CT, 136. *See also* Children's Seashore House; Crawford Allen Hospital; Sea Breeze Hospital
How the Other Half Lives (Riis), 83
Hudak, Edward John, 120–21

immigrant children, 15, 23–24
immigrants: ocean passage, 35
incubator exhibits, 39, 66
industrialization, 3, 140
infant mortality, 13–14, 29, 88; milk purity and, 82, 83

Jones, Helen Lois, 24

Kelley, Florence, 18, 21
Koch, Robert, 16, 40, 130

Last Child in the Woods (Louv), 147–48
light therapy. *See* sunlight and sunbathing; UV lamps
Little Women (Alcott), 97
Lord Mayor Treloar Cripples' Home and Cottage, 52
Louv, Richard: *Last Child in the Woods*, 147–48

Marion, Joe ("Smiling Joe"), 39–40, 112–17, *113*
Massachusetts Emergency and Hygiene Association, 18, 33
miasma theory of disease, 3, 53
middle class, 12, 17, 59, 94, 103, 108, 110;

families, 65, 69, 80, 95; mothers, 22
milk: purity and impurity, 82–84, 88; vitamin-supplemented, 135
mothers: at Children's Seashore House, 79–82, 84–87; and day care, 92–93; middle-class, 22; pressures on, 82–84; and seaside benefits, 88–91; working class, 22–23, 28, 31, 34, 93–96

neonatal care, 39, 66
neurasthenia, 16, 104
Newark, NJ, 38
New York Association for Improving the Condition of the Poor, 26
New York City, 31; "breathing space" in, 26; Central Park, 20, 61; child and infant mortality in, 14, 17; floating hospitals of, 26, 31; *Forty-Two Kids*, *100*, 100; Fresh Air Fund of, 26, 31; population of, 13; sand gardens of, 19; Seaside Hospital of, 89; street play in, 17, 21; tenement apartments in, 83. *See also* Association for Improving the Condition of the Poor; Coney Island
nosology, 14
Nyack, NY, 32–33

ocean air, 43, 49, 53–54
ocean bathing, 50–52, 64, 70–73
Oliver, George, 41–43, 44
Olmsted, Frederick Law, 19, 61
orthopedics, 47–48, 102, *111*, 111, *113*, 113–14
Osborne, Richard, 60–61
Ovington, Earle, 76–77
ozone, 53, 54, 57

Packard, John H., 71, 73, 146
parks, 19, 20, 21–22
Pasteur, Louis, 38, 40
pediatrics, formalization of, 38
Philadelphia, 9–10, 13–14, 27–29, 31, 104; Atlantic City and, 60–61, 63, 90, 105, 118; child and infant mortality in, 14, 29; Children's Country Week Association of, 26; children's hospitals in, 25, 42, 147; home health conditions in, 23–25; immigrant children in, 23–24; parks in, 20; Starr Centre Association of, 90; Windmill Island near, 27–28
phototherapy, 54–56, *125*, 126–29, *128*, 134–41, 150; with UV lamps, 7, 54, 123–26, 129–37, 141
Pitney, Jonathan, 58, 60
play, 20–21, 116; street, 17, 21, 22
playgrounds, 19, 20, 21
plumbing systems, 82, 83
polio, 3, 110, 120, 145
pollution, air, xii, 15, 22, 136
Pott's disease, 14, 139
public health, xi, 3, 13, 53, 139, 149–50. *See also* home health conditions; sanitation, urban

rabies, 38, 40
race, 74, 94; "betterment," 19, 56; rickets and, 15
railroads, 34, 59, 60, 61, 62, 63, 65, 79, 80
Red Bank Sanitarium (New Jersey), 9–10, 28–29, 31
Reed, Boardman, 44, 46, 53
rheumatoid endocarditis, 118
rickets, 15, 21, 110; light therapy for, 123, *124*, 134, 135; vitamin D therapy for, 135
Riis, Jacob: *How the Other Half Lives*, 83
Robison, John, 42
Rollier, Auguste, 54, 55, 126, 130, 133, 141
rolling chairs: Atlantic City, 72, 73–76
Roosevelt, Theodore, 114

Salt in My Soul (Smith), 144, 151
sandboxes, 18–19
sand gardens, 18, 19
Sanitarium Association of Philadelphia, 9–11, 27, 33
sanitation, urban, 3, 15, 17
sanitoriums, 26, 27–28; in Belgium, 147; in Red Bank, NJ, 9–10, 28–29, 31; in Waterford, CT, 136

Schwartz, Plato, 136, 137
scrofula, 14, 41, 44, 45, 139
sea air, 43, 49, 53–54
Sea-Air and Sea-Bathing for Children and Invalids (Brochard), 41
sea-bathing, 50–52, 64, 70–73
Sea Breeze Hospital (Coney Island, New York City), 26–27, 39–40, 47, 48, 66, 68, 80, 111–17; sunbathing at, 126, *128*
Seaside Hospital (New York City), 89
Seaside Sanatorium (Waterford, (CT), 136
sea voyages, 35, 36, 77
seawater, 49–52, 57; cystic fibrosis and, 143–44
Singer, Charles I., 145–46
"Smiling Joe." *See* Marion, Joe ("Smiling Joe")
Smith, Lawrence, 123, *124*
Smith, Mallory: *Salt in My Soul*, 144, 151
social class. *See* middle class; upper class; working class
social workers, 23–24, 25, 32, 104
spas and health resorts, 26, 34, 146–47
Stafford, Jane, 145
Stainthorpe, Helen, 86–87
suffragists, 75
summer camps, 43, 108–11
sunlamps. *See* UV lamps
sunlight and sunbathing, 54–56, *125*, 126–29, *128*, 134–41, 150
swimming, 108; in the East River, 100; in the ocean, 1, 48, 50, 68, 71. *See also* balneotherapy
Switzerland, 55, 133, 136

tanning and tanned skin, 139–40
tenements, xii, 21, 26, 83
traffic accidents, 17–18
tuberculosis (TB): bone, 40, 132; and Children's Seashore House, 43, 92, 110; heliotherapy and UV therapy and, 127–28, 130–31, 132, 133, 136; Joe Marion and, 39–40, 112–17; mountain travel and, 36; pediatric, 14–15, 16, 21, 44–45, 47, 115; Pott's disease, 14, 139; sanitariums and, 26; scrofula, 14, 41, 44, 45, 139; sea air and, 53; sea-bathing therapy for, 52; and Sea Breeze Hospital, 39–40, 48, 115; skin, 130–31, 132, 133

"ugly laws," 18
ultraviolet (UV) rays, 54, 57, 130, 136, 150. *See also* UV lamps
Unger, Lester, 134, 135
upper class, 12, 17, 81, 106, 110
US Children's Bureau, 84, 139–40, 141
UV lamps, 7, 54, 123–26, 129–37, 141; at Cincinnati General Hospital, 137

vacations, 36, 59; prescribed, 145–46
Velveteen Rabbit, The (Williams), 97

wheelchairs, 65, 73, 74
Willard, DeForest, 45, 131, 132–33
working class: children, 24, 26, 28–29, 105–6, 110, 121–22; and day care, 92–93; families, 25, 26, 31–32, 59–60, 65, 82, 83; mothers, 22–23, 28, 31, 34, 82–84, 88–91, 93–96

Young Men's Christian Association (YMCA), 108

Zakrzewska, Marie, 18
Zueblin, Charles, 19–20

WEYERHAEUSER ENVIRONMENTAL BOOKS

The Beach Cure: A History of Healing on Northeastern Shores, by Meghan Crnic
Contaminated Country: Nuclear Colonialism and Aboriginal Resistance in Australia, by Jessica Urwin
Animating Central Park: A Multispecies History, by Dawn Day Biehler
Cleaning Up the Bomb Factory: Grassroots Activism and Nuclear Waste in the Midwest, by Casey A. Huegel
Capturing Glaciers: A History of Repeat Photography and Global Warming, by Dani Inkpen
The Toxic Ship: The Voyage of the Khian Sea *and the Global Waste Trade*, by Simone M. Müller
People of the Ecotone: Environment and Indigenous Power at the Center of Early America, by Robert Michael Morrissey
Charged: A History of Batteries and Lessons for a Clean Energy Future, by James Morton Turner
Wetlands in a Dry Land: More-Than-Human Histories of Australia's Murray-Darling Basin, by Emily O'Gorman
Seeds of Control: Japan's Empire of Forestry in Colonial Korea, by David Fedman
Fir and Empire: The Transformation of Forests in Early Modern China, by Ian M. Miller
Communist Pigs: An Animal History of East Germany's Rise and Fall, by Thomas Fleischman
Footprints of War: Militarized Landscapes in Vietnam, by David Biggs
Cultivating Nature: The Conservation of a Valencian Working Landscape, by Sarah R. Hamilton
Bringing Whales Ashore: Oceans and the Environment of Early Modern Japan, by Jakobina K. Arch
The Organic Profit: Rodale and the Making of Marketplace Environmentalism, by Andrew N. Case
Seismic City: An Environmental History of San Francisco's 1906 Earthquake, by Joanna L. Dyl
Smell Detectives: An Olfactory History of Nineteenth-Century Urban America, by Melanie A. Kiechle
Defending Giants: The Redwood Wars and the Transformation of American Environmental Politics, by Darren Frederick Speece
The City Is More Than Human: An Animal History of Seattle, by Frederick L. Brown
Wilderburbs: Communities on Nature's Edge, by Lincoln Bramwell
How to Read the American West: A Field Guide, by William Wyckoff
Behind the Curve: Science and the Politics of Global Warming, by Joshua P. Howe
Whales and Nations: Environmental Diplomacy on the High Seas, by Kurkpatrick Dorsey

Loving Nature, Fearing the State: Environmentalism and Antigovernment Politics before Reagan, by Brian Allen Drake
Pests in the City: Flies, Bedbugs, Cockroaches, and Rats, by Dawn Day Biehler
Tangled Roots: The Appalachian Trail and American Environmental Politics, by Sarah Mittlefehldt
Vacationland: Tourism and Environment in the Colorado High Country, by William Philpott
Car Country: An Environmental History, by Christopher W. Wells
Nature Next Door: Cities and Trees in the American Northeast, by Ellen Stroud
Pumpkin: The Curious History of an American Icon, by Cindy Ott
The Promise of Wilderness: American Environmental Politics since 1964, by James Morton Turner
The Republic of Nature: An Environmental History of the United States, by Mark Fiege
A Storied Wilderness: Rewilding the Apostle Islands, by James W. Feldman
Iceland Imagined: Nature, Culture, and Storytelling in the North Atlantic, by Karen Oslund
Quagmire: Nation-Building and Nature in the Mekong Delta, by David Biggs
Seeking Refuge: Birds and Landscapes of the Pacific Flyway, by Robert M. Wilson
Toxic Archipelago: A History of Industrial Disease in Japan, by Brett L. Walker
Dreaming of Sheep in Navajo Country, by Marsha L. Weisiger
Shaping the Shoreline: Fisheries and Tourism on the Monterey Coast, by Connie Y. Chiang
The Fishermen's Frontier: People and Salmon in Southeast Alaska, by David F. Arnold
Making Mountains: New York City and the Catskills, by David Stradling
Plowed Under: Agriculture and Environment in the Palouse, by Andrew P. Duffin
The Country in the City: The Greening of the San Francisco Bay Area, by Richard A. Walker
Native Seattle: Histories from the Crossing-Over Place, by Coll Thrush
Drawing Lines in the Forest: Creating Wilderness Areas in the Pacific Northwest, by Kevin R. Marsh
Public Power, Private Dams: The Hells Canyon High Dam Controversy, by Karl Boyd Brooks
Windshield Wilderness: Cars, Roads, and Nature in Washington's National Parks, by David Louter
On the Road Again: Montana's Changing Landscape, by William Wyckoff
Wilderness Forever: Howard Zahniser and the Path to the Wilderness Act, by Mark Harvey
The Lost Wolves of Japan, by Brett L. Walker
Landscapes of Conflict: The Oregon Story, 1940–2000, by William G. Robbins
Faith in Nature: Environmentalism as Religious Quest, by Thomas R. Dunlap
The Nature of Gold: An Environmental History of the Klondike Gold Rush, by Kathryn Morse

Where Land and Water Meet: A Western Landscape Transformed, by Nancy Langston
The Rhine: An Eco-Biography, 1815–2000, by Mark Cioc
Driven Wild: How the Fight against Automobiles Launched the Modern Wilderness Movement, by Paul S. Sutter
George Perkins Marsh: Prophet of Conservation, by David Lowenthal
Making Salmon: An Environmental History of the Northwest Fisheries Crisis, by Joseph E. Taylor III
Irrigated Eden: The Making of an Agricultural Landscape in the American West, by Mark Fiege
The Dawn of Conservation Diplomacy: U.S.-Canadian Wildlife Protection Treaties in the Progressive Era, by Kurkpatrick Dorsey
Landscapes of Promise: The Oregon Story, 1800–1940, by William G. Robbins
Forest Dreams, Forest Nightmares: The Paradox of Old Growth in the Inland West, by Nancy Langston
The Natural History of Puget Sound Country, by Arthur R. Kruckeberg

Weyerhaeuser Environmental Classics

Debating Malthus: A Documentary Reader on Population, Resources, and the Environment, edited by Robert J. Mayhew
Environmental Justice in Postwar America: A Documentary Reader, edited by Christopher W. Wells
Making Climate Change History: Documents from Global Warming's Past, edited by Joshua P. Howe
Nuclear Reactions: Documenting American Encounters with Nuclear Energy, edited by James W. Feldman
The Wilderness Writings of Howard Zahniser, edited by Mark Harvey
The Environmental Moment: 1968–1972, edited by David Stradling
Reel Nature: America's Romance with Wildlife on Film, by Gregg Mitman
DDT, Silent Spring, *and the Rise of Environmentalism,* edited by Thomas R. Dunlap
Conservation in the Progressive Era: Classic Texts, edited by David Stradling
Man and Nature: Or, Physical Geography as Modified by Human Action, by George Perkins Marsh
A Symbol of Wilderness: Echo Park and the American Conservation Movement, by Mark W. T. Harvey
Tutira: The Story of a New Zealand Sheep Station, by Herbert Guthrie-Smith
Mountain Gloom and Mountain Glory: The Development of the Aesthetics of the Infinite, by Marjorie Hope Nicolson
The Great Columbia Plain: A Historical Geography, 1805–1910, by Donald W. Meinig

Cycle of Fire

Fire: A Brief History, second edition, by Stephen J. Pyne
The Ice: A Journey to Antarctica, by Stephen J. Pyne
Burning Bush: A Fire History of Australia, by Stephen J. Pyne
Fire in America: A Cultural History of Wildland and Rural Fire, by Stephen J. Pyne
Vestal Fire: An Environmental History, Told through Fire, of Europe and Europe's Encounter with the World, by Stephen J. Pyne
World Fire: The Culture of Fire on Earth, by Stephen J. Pyne

Also available:

Awful Splendour: A Fire History of Canada, by Stephen J. Pyne